MW01492947

Prescription Drugs
and Their Side Effects

by Edward L. Stern

This edition was compiled and edited by
Elza Dinwiddie-Boyd

A Perigee Book

Perigee Books
are published by
The Putnam Publishing Group
200 Madison Avenue
New York, NY 10016

Library of Congress Cataloging-in-Publication Data

Stern, Edward L.
Prescription drugs and their side effects / by Edward L. Stern.
p. cm.
''This edition was compiled and edited by Elza Dinwiddie-Boyd.''
''A Perigee book.''
Includes indexes.
ISBN 0-399-51641-7
1. Drugs—Side effects—Handbooks, manuals, etc. I. Dinwiddie,
Elza Teresa. II. Title.
RM302.5.S75   1991   90-39508 CIP
615'.7042—dc20

Printed in the United States of America

1   2   3   4   5   6   7   8   9   10

This book is printed on acid-free paper.

CONTENTS

Prescription Drugs and Their Side Effects

is an analysis of the 396 most frequently prescribed drugs as tabulated by the New York State Pharmacy Board, The National Prescription Audit, and various other listings and tabulations.

Additional research conducted by Nayyar Imam, R.Ph.

INTRODUCTION

Why This Book

What prompts a layman to write a book about the side effects and adverse reactions to prescription drugs?

After all, I'm not a physician, a medical researcher, a pharmacist, or an employee of a drug company.

But I am a father. A son. A husband. I have taken prescription drugs from time to time, and I have friends and relatives who have. Most of us do.

During an eighteen-month period, individuals close to me experienced the following disturbing medical problems: My son was rushed to the hospital with a severe penicillin reaction. My mother was hospitalized after she blacked out. A cousin confided that he thought he had become impotent. And my best friend's wife was taken off "the pill" because of an assortment of medical difficulties. In each instance, after much heartache, pain, and costly medical care, the problem was diagnosed as a reaction to a particular drug.

And so I decided to write this book to *alert* consumers to the *possible* side effects of and adverse reactions to the prescription drugs they take. Side effects and reactions such as:

dizziness, dry mouth, stomach cramps, loss of balance, bleeding, fluid retention, headaches, vomiting, fever, rash, nausea, loss of appetite, itching, diarrhea, blurred vision, pains in the joints, impotence, insomnia, jitters, fluttering, constipation, shortness of breath, drowsiness, depression

After all, if you know *in advance* the possible reactions you may encounter as a result of taking a particular drug, you'll be prepared for any health changes you experience—whether slight or pronounced—and you'll also be able to describe any unusual side effects to your own physician.

One simple example of the needless confusion, discomfort, and cost that result from taking medication without knowing all its possible effects is illustrated in the following case.

5

A woman I know had been taking a blood pressure medication for more than a year. During this time, she was constantly bothered by a stuffy nose. She spent hundreds of dollars and many hours in doctors' offices seeking a remedy for her stuffy nose. The stuffy nose was a side effect associated with her blood pressure medication. But, unfortunately, she never connected the two. And she never mentioned the stuffy nose to the family physician who prescribed the blood pressure medication. In this age of specialization, she took her nose problem to a "nose specialist." Her discomfort probably could have been eased immediately if she had been able to connect the cause and effect to the prescription drug she was taking.

How We Determined Which Drugs to Include

An article in *The New York Times* estimated that more than *one billion* drug prescriptions are written by doctors in the United States each year. Chances are that you or someone in your family is taking at least one prescription drug *right now!* Just look in your medicine cabinet. If you're an average consumer, you've probably had one or more prescriptions filled in the last thirty days.

Each month Americans purchase millions of sleeping pills, tranquilizers, diuretics, blood pressure medicines, birth control pills, decongestants, antihistamines, antidepressants, pain relievers, antibiotics, anticoagulants, weight control pills, hormones, and anticonvulsants.

We take drugs to make us feel better. To end discomfort. To stop pain. To induce sleep. To increase energy. To fight infection.

Often these drugs bring about an assortment of side effects in susceptible individuals. Since there are thousands of different prescription medicines on the market, I was faced with the problem of determining which drugs to include in the book and which to omit.

One day I was having a prescription filled at our local druggist's and noticed a large price list posted at the end of his counter. It listed the *most frequently prescribed* prescription drugs as tabulated by the New York State Pharmacy Board. I had my answer. The book would include these drugs plus other popular prescription medications (360 in all) culled from various sources and would, therefore, help the greatest number of people possible without being padded with thousands of obscure drugs. My goal was to produce a volume inexpensive enough so that every consumer could afford a copy. Therefore, there may be some drugs that have been prescribed for you or your family that are *not* included in this volume. Don't be bashful. If you're concerned about the possible side effects of a drug you take that's not listed here, ask your physician to supply you with the information from his or her own reference material. There is a section at the end of this book for special notes. Use it to add specific information relating to your family's prescription medicines.

The intention of this book is to tell consumers . . .

1. the reason a particular drug is usually *prescribed* . . .
2. the *precautions* to observe when taking this drug . . .
3. the possible *side effects* and *adverse reactions* that may occur when taking the drug.

It should be pointed out that side effects and adverse reactions occur *only* in susceptible individuals. Most persons who take prescription drugs experience few, if any, side effects or adverse reactions. A particular drug has been prescribed because, in the opinion of the physician, the benefits far outweigh any risk.

In addition to the above, this volume also includes:

• The generic name of each drug. If your family physician will prescribe by the generic name whenever possible, you'll be able to save money on almost every prescription you fill.

• The name of the pharmaceutical company that makes the drug.

• The form the drug comes in (tablet, solution, capsule, drops, creams, etc.).

• The available strengths of the drug.

• The route for taking the drug (oral, intravaginal, rectal, intranasal, ophthalmic, etc.).

• An easy-to-follow A–Z index.

• Space for you and your physician to make special notes about your particular medication.

How the Information Was Compiled

First, we edited into easy-to-understand language the information contained in the package folders sent by drug companies to physicians and pharmacists along with the drugs. Next, we verified this information, drug by drug, against the most recent *Physician's Desk Reference* (PDR), plus modifications from PDR supplements.

In researching this book, my major concern was to keep it an easy-to-use, uncomplicated reference source. Therefore, I *have not* included every possible drug form and dosage strength available for each of the 360 drugs. I have, however, listed those forms and strengths that are the most common. In addition, I have excluded, in all cases, forms of any drug that are injected, since this procedure is not usually left in the hands of the consumer.

Thirty-six of the drugs appear under their generic names. These are: Acetaminophen with Codeine, Amitriptyline HCl, Amoxicillin, Allopurinol, Ampicillin, Chlordiazepoxide, Diazepam, Dicloxacillin, Digoxin, Dipyridamole, Doxycline, Erythromycin, Folic acid, Furosemide, Hydralazine, Hydrochlorothiazide, Hydrocortisone, Hydroxyzine HCl, Ibuprofen, Isorbide Dinitrate, Imipramine HCl, Lithium Carbonate, Meclizine, Meprobamate, Metronidazole, Nitroglycerin, Nystatin, Penicillin-V Potassium, Phenobarbital, Potassium Chloride, Prednisone, Propranalol, Tetracycline, Thyroid, Triamcinolone Acetonide, Trimethoprim with Sulfamethoxazole. In the alphabetical listings of these drugs, we have included the form and dosage strengths that are *most frequently prescribed*. Had we tried to include every form and every strength available for each generic drug, the book would have become confusing and unwieldy since most drugs are produced by dozens of different manufacturers in a multitude of dosage forms and strengths.

A Note on Ordering Drugs Generically

State laws have been passed which permit a pharmacist to fill a prescription generically. Simply stated, this means that a pharmacist may stock a brand of drug which is identical to the one your physician has prescribed but less expensive. If your physician gives his permission on the prescription form, the pharmacist may substitute less expensive brands of the drug. This will occur most often if the drug is a single chemical and not a combination. For example, your physician may prescribe a specific brand of tetracycline for an infection. You take your prescription to a large pharmacy that is part of a national chain. This pharmacy carries its own brand of tetracycline, which is less expensive than the brand prescribed. If your physician has indicated on the form that the prescription may be filled generically, your pharmacist must substitute the less expensive house brand. This results in a saving to you.

It is possible that your physician does not wish a generic substitution to be made even though one is possible. If he so indicates on the prescription form, your pharmacist cannot make the substitution.

To find out if you can save money, talk with your physician to determine if the prescription drug you are taking can be replaced with a less expensive brand.

A Few Words of Caution

This book is not intended to be used in any way for self-medication. Prescription drugs should be taken *only* under the supervision of a licensed physician.

In prescribing a drug, your physician is aware of the possible hazards associated with the drug and of how these may affect you. Therefore, you should *never* take any medication that has been prescribed for someone else. Various drugs affect different people in different ways.

Drugs taken in combination may produce side effects not noted when either drug is taken alone. Always inform a physician or dentist of every drug you are taking or have taken in the past. Never mix drugs unless you are so directed by a physician, and always adhere strictly to the prescribed dosage.

Most drugs are not recommended during pregnancy; pregnant women and women who plan to become pregnant should be particularly cautious, and should inform any physician treating them of their pregnancy or intended pregnancy.

The side effects and adverse reactions listed here are those the drug companies *are aware of* based upon their own research plus feedback received from physicians, pharmacists, and consumers. We have included *only the most common ones*—those that the patient himself can easily identify. However, just because a side effect is not listed here *does not mean that it may not be caused by the drug.* If at any time while taking a particular medication, you experience anything abnormal, *consult your physician immediately.* It is his responsibility to determine if the side effect is tolerable in light of the therapeutic value of the drug.

In the DOSAGE section, we have included *the most commonly prescribed dosage strengths of each drug.*

Under WHEN PRESCRIBED, the common intended use for the drug (i.e., that ailment for which it is most commonly prescribed) has been listed. It may be possible that in certain cases a drug has been prescribed for some other condition or ailment. Also, since all drugs include the general phrase "Persons with known hypersensitivity to [drug name] should not use this drug," we have often omitted the phrase. For example, many drugs contain pure aspirin and these should be used with caution by people with known hypersensitivity to aspirin and related compounds.

The following adverse reactions have been reported in users of oral contraceptives: changes in sex drive, changes in appetite, headache, nervousness, dizziness, fatigue, backache, increase in facial hair, loss of scalp hair, skin eruptions, itching. However, an association between the symptoms and the use of oral contraceptives has been neither confirmed nor disproved. See individual entries for specific details.

In the SIDE EFFECTS AND ADVERSE REACTIONS section, the following entry appears for all antibiotics, "superinfection by nonsusceptible organism." This indicates that a particular infection may be caused by a reinfection by the original organism, which has developed resistance to the antibiotic. Therefore, if you do not obtain relief in a short period of time, be sure to consult your physician.

Remember, your physician is the final authority on the drug he has prescribed. His instructions, even if different from those contained in this book, should be followed.

Prescription Drugs and Their Side Effects was written for you. Your family. Your friends. It was written for you to use. To help you know what changes *may* be taking place in your own mind and body. To enable you to ask your physician intelligent questions and to *explain* certain symptoms more clearly. It is not a book for doctors or pharmacists. It is not intended to be an encyclopedia listing every conceivable side effect. It was not developed as a pharmacological tome or as the last word in drug information. Every individual is different, and drugs affect people in different ways. It is, however, designed to be an easy-to-follow, basic reference source for consumers written in easy-to-understand language. Listing each of the 396 drugs in alphabetical order, the book is intentionally devoid of subjective text material. There is no attempt to *evaluate* any drug listed.

FOREWORD

The 6th edition of *Prescription Drugs and Their Side Effects* is revised and expanded to include 396 of the most frequently prescribed drugs. The dynamic nature of the pharmaceutical industry requires regular updating of this volume. For example, a new product, Voltaren®, is listed on the National Prescription Audit as the 161st most frequently prescribed drug in 1988. In 1989 Voltaren is number 25. In contrast to this increase, other medications have shown a sharp decrease in frequency. This edition represents our effort to keep abreast of these changes in prescription patterns.

The new entries are clustered around antihypertensives, antibiotics, antiarthritics, oral contraceptives and serum-cholesterol-lowering agents. The new entries are taken from the 500 most frequently prescribed drugs. We have also deleted a product recently taken off the market and inserted new indications for others.

It should be noted that the first treatment of choice for lowering high levels of serum cholesterol is dietary restrictions and that manufacturers of oral contraceptives issue a strong precaution against cigarette smoking.

The 6th edition has retained the easy-to-follow, plain-English, basic-reference quality of the previous editions.

We wish to thank Elza Dinwiddie-Boyd and Patricia Rose Curtis, R.Ph. for helping to make this latest edition possible.

THE EDITORS

ALPHABETICAL DESCRIPTION OF 396 DRUGS

ACCUTANE® (Roche Laboratories)

Generic Name: Isotretinoin

Dosage Form	Strength	Route
Capsule	10 mg	Oral
	20 mg	Oral
	40 mg	Oral

When Prescribed: Accutane is prescribed for the treatment of acne. Because of significant adverse effects associated with its use, Accutane is prescribed only for those patients with severe acne who do not respond to conventional therapy, including antibiotics.

Precautions and Warnings: Accutane must not be used by females who are pregnant or who intend to become pregnant while undergoing treatment. Accutane is a powerful and effective drug.

Side Effects and Adverse Reactions: Headache, nausea, vomiting, visual disturbance, inflammation of the lips, inflammation of the conjunctiva (part of the eye), rash, thinning of hair, skin infection, fatigue, change in skin pigment, weight loss, inflammation of gums, abnormal menstruation, dry eyes, decrease in night vision, depression, dizziness, weakness, insomnia, lethargy.

ACETAMINOPHEN WITH CODEINE

The generic name for a drug produced by numerous companies.

Dosage Form	Strength	Route
Tablet	No. 1	Oral
	No. 2	Oral
	No. 3	Oral
	No. 4	Oral

When Prescribed: Acetaminophen with codeine is prescribed for relief of pain of various causes and for relief of aches.

Precautions and Warnings: Acetaminophen with codeine contains a narcotic pain reliever which may be habit forming. This preparation may cause drowsiness. Therefore, driving motor vehicles or operating dangerous machinery is discouraged while taking this medicine.

Side Effects and Adverse Reactions: Drowsiness, constipation, nausea, lightheadedness, dizziness, vomiting, mood changes, itching, rash.

ACHROMYCIN® V (Lederle Laboratories)

Generic Name: Tetracycline HCl

Dosage Form	Strength	Route
Capsule	100 mg	Oral
	250 mg	Oral
	500 mg	Oral
Syrup	125 mg/5cc	Oral

When Prescribed: Achromycin is an effective antibiotic prescribed for many different types of infection. It is often used in place of penicillin in patients allergic to penicillin. The length of therapy depends on the type of ailment being treated.

Precautions and Warnings: Achromycin should not be taken by persons overly sensitive to tetracycline. Not recommended for pregnant women, infants or children under the age of 8.

Side Effects and Adverse Reactions: Exaggerated sunburn can occur while taking this drug. As with other antibiotics, organisms that are not susceptible to its actions may grow. This is known as superinfection. If this occurs, the use of Achromycin should be discontinued. The following adverse reactions have been reported: loss of appetite, nausea, vomiting, diarrhea, inflammation of the tongue, difficulty swallowing, stomachache, inflammation of bowel and genital region, skin rash, hives, swelling, shock, discoloration of growing teeth.

ACTIFED®WITH CODEINE COUGH SYRUP (Burroughs Wellcome Company)

Generic Name: Codeine phosphate, triprolidine hydrochloride, pseudoephedrine hydrochloride

Dosage Form	Strength	Route
Liquid	Available in one strength only	Oral

When Prescribed: Actifed cough syrup is prescribed for the relief of cough in conditions such as the common cold, acute bronchitis, asthma, breathing difficulties (croup), and emphysema.

Precautions and Warnings: Should be used with caution in patients with high blood pressure. A low incidence of drowsiness has been reported. Therefore, Actifed should not be taken before undertaking a task requiring complete alertness. Actifed contains codeine, which may be habit forming.

Side Effects and Adverse Reactions: Mild stimulation, mild sedation (drowsiness).

ADAPIN® (Pennwalt Pharmaceutical Division)

Generic Name: Doxepin HCl

Dosage Form	Strength	Route
Capsule	10 mg	Oral
	25 mg	
	50 mg	
	75 mg	
	100 mg	

When Prescribed: Adapin is prescribed to relieve anxiety and/or depression in patients with various kinds of mental or emotional problems.

Precautions and Warnings: The safe use of this drug in children under 12 years of age, pregnant women, or nursing mothers has not been established. Adapin should not be taken with alcohol, tranquilizers, sedatives, or sleeping pills without your physician's consent. If drowsiness occurs you should not drive or operate dangerous machinery.

Side Effects and Adverse Reactions: Dry mouth, blurred vision, constipation, drowsiness, rapid heartbeat, abnormal movements, increased sweating, weakness, dizziness, fatigue, weight gain, swelling, abnormal sensations, flushing, chills, ringing in the ears, increased sensitivity to light, decreased sex drive, rash, itching.

ADIPEX-P® (Lemmon Company)

Generic Name: Phentermine hydrochloride

Dosage Form	Strength	Route
Tablet	37.5 mg	Oral

When Prescribed: Adipex-P is prescribed for the management of obesity in a regimen of weight reduction based on caloric restriction.

Precautions and Warnings: Adipex-P should be avoided by patients with high blood pressure, hyperthyroidism, and glaucoma. It should also be avoided by patients with a history of drug abuse and during or within 14 days following the administration of monoamine oxidase (MAO) inhibitors (a group of drugs used to treat depression). No study has been conducted so far concerning the use of this drug in pregnancy. Adipex-P is not recommended for use by children under 12. If a patient is using insulin, she or he should inform the physician before starting this drug.

Side Effects and Adverse Reactions: Elevation of blood pressure, increase in heart rate, restlessness, dizziness, trouble sleeping, headache, dryness of mouth, unpleasant taste, diarrhea, constipation, impotence, convulsions.

ALDACTAZIDE® (Searle and Company)

Generic Name: Spironolactone with hydrochlorothiazide

Dosage Form	Strength	Route
Tablet	25 mg	
	50 mg	Oral

When Prescribed: Aldactazide is prescribed for treatment of high blood pressure, water accumulation due to congestive heart failure, cirrhosis of the liver, kidney disease and water retention of unknown cause. This preparation is a combination of two drugs which help the kidneys to pass water and salt and help reduce the symptoms of the above-mentioned conditions. Aldactazide is usually not prescribed initially, but only after your physician has determined that the fixed combination of drugs will be proper for you.

Precautions and Warnings: This is a potent drug which requires close supervision by your physician. Your physician should be consulted if any of the symptoms listed below appear.

Side Effects and Adverse Reactions: Dryness of mouth, thirst, drowsiness, tiredness, mental confusion, diarrhea, intestinal cramps, development of breasts in males, loss of sexual drive, masculinizing traits in females (including beard growth, deepening of voice and menstrual irregularities), headache, skin eruptions, hives, fever, loss of balance, abnormal bruising, loss of appetite, nausea, vomiting, rash, itching, abnormal skin sensation (including tingling, crawling and burning), yellowing of skin, yellow appearance of objects (yellow vi-

ALDACTONE® (Searle and Company)

Generic Name: Spironolactone

Dosage Form	Strength	Route
Tablet	25 mg	Oral
	100 mg	Oral

When Prescribed: Aldactone causes increased amounts of sodium and water to be passed from the body (diuresis). It is prescribed to lower blood pressure. It can also be prescribed for water accumulation resistant to other diuretic therapy. Aldactone is one of the constituents in Aldactazide (see previous entry) and is used to treat the same symptoms. Your physician has determined which of these drugs (Aldactone or Aldactazide) is best for your particular case.

Precautions and Warnings: Your physician should be consulted if any of the symptoms listed below appears.

Side Effects and Adverse Reactions: Dryness of mouth, thirst, drowsiness, tiredness, mental confusion, headache, diarrhea, intestinal cramps, development of breasts in males, loss of sexual drive, masculinizing traits in females (including beard growth, deepening of the voice and menstrual irregularities), skin eruptions, hives, fever, loss of balance.

Aldactazide-(Continued)

sion), increased reactivity to sunlight, muscle spasms, weakness and restlessness, sore throat, sores in the mouth.

ALDOMET® (Merck Sharp and Dohme)

Generic Name: Methyldopa

Dosage Form	Strength	Route
Tablet	125 mg	Oral
	250 mg	Oral
	500 mg	Oral

When Prescribed: Aldomet is usually prescribed for lowering blood pressure in patients with sustained moderate to severe high blood pressure (hypertension). Unlike most drugs which lower blood pressure, Aldomet exerts its action via the nervous system.

Precautions and Warnings: Aldomet is a potent drug that is not recommended for mild cases of high blood pressure.

Side Effects and Adverse Reactions: Sedation, headache and weakness. Lowering of blood pressure (the intended effect of the drug) may cause dizziness, lightheadedness and fainting. Other adverse reactions include slowing of the heart, nasal congestion, dryness of the mouth, constipation, gas, diarrhea, nausea, vomiting, sore tongue, blackening of tongue, swollen glands in neck, weight gain, water retention, breast enlargement, lactation, impotence, loss of sexual drive, skin rash, pain in joints and muscles, skin discomfort, shaking or tremors, nightmares, mental depression, darkening of urine after voiding, fever.

ALDORIL® (Merck Sharp and Dohme)

Generic Name: Methyldopa, hydrochlorothiazide

Dosage Form	Strength	Route
Tablet	15 mg	Oral
	25 mg	Oral

When Prescribed: Aldoril is a combination of two drugs prescribed for the control of high blood pressure especially in cases where water and salt retention is a problem. Aldoril is usually not prescribed initially after a diagnosis of high blood pressure but only when your physician has determined that the fixed combination of drugs in Aldoril is the proper dosage for you.

Precautions and Warnings: Aldoril is a potent drug which should only be taken under close supervision of your physician. Periodic blood and other tests should be done while taking Aldoril. Mothers should not nurse while taking Aldoril.

Side Effects and Adverse Reactions: Sleepiness, headache, weakness, dizziness, lightheadedness, numbness or tingling of skin, tremors, spasms, nightmares, depression, nausea, vomiting, constipation, gas, diarrhea, dryness of mouth, blackened tongue, fever, nasal congestion, breast enlargement, impotence, decreased sex drive, rash, loss of appetite, stomach irritation, cramps, blurred vision, slowing of heart rate, dryness of mouth, weight gain, water retention, skin discomfort, shaking or tremors, nightmares, depression, soreness of tongue.

ALLOPURINOL The generic name of a drug produced by numerous companies in different strengths. Also marketed as:
LOPURIN® Boots
ZYLOPRIM® Burroughs Wellcome

Dosage Form	Strength	Route
Tablet	100 mg	Oral
	300 mg	Oral

When Prescribed: Allopurinol is prescribed for patients with signs and symptoms of gout. It is also given to patients who are receiving cancer therapy.

Precautions and Warnings: An increase in acute attacks of gout has been reported during the early stages of allopurinol administration. A sufficient amount of fluid intake is necessary with allopurinol therapy. The first sign of skin rash should be reported to the physician.

Side Effects and Adverse Reactions: Diarrhea, nausea, skin rash, fever, headache, abdominal pain, dyspepsia.

ALUPENT® (Boehringer Ingelheim Ltd.)

Generic Name: Metaproterenol sulfate

Dosage Form	Strength	Route
Tablet	10 mg	Oral
	20 mg	
Metered dose inhaler	15 ml	Inhaled orally
Syrup	10 mg/5 ml	Oral
Inhalant solution	5%	Inhaled orally

When Prescribed: Alupent is prescribed for the relief of breathing difficulties associated with bronchial asthma, bronchitis, or emphysema.

Precautions and Warnings: Consult your physician if the prescribed dosage does not provide relief. Do not exceed the prescribed dosage. The inhaled forms of this drug are not recommended for use in children under 12 years of age. The tablets are not recommended for children under 6 years of age.

Side Effects and Adverse Reactions: Nervousness, rapid heart rate, tremor, nausea, elevated blood pressure, heart flutters, vomiting, bad taste.

AMBENYL® COUGH SYRUP (Marion Laboratories, Inc.)

Generic Name: Codeine phosphate, bromodiphenhydramine hydrochloride, alcohol

Dosage Form	Strength	Route
Liquid	Available in one strength only	Oral

When Prescribed: Ambenyl is prescribed for coughs accompanying colds and coughs accompanying allergies. The main effects of the drug are (1) reduction of frequency of coughing, (2) thinning of mucus for easier expectoration (passing from respiratory tract).

Precautions and Warnings: Ambenyl causes drowsiness in some people. Patients who become drowsy should not drive vehicles or engage in activities requiring alert responses. Sleeping pills, sedatives, alcohol, or tranquilizers should not be used with Ambenyl. Ambenyl contains codeine, which may be habit forming. This drug may inhibit milk production in nursing mothers.

Side Effects and Adverse Reactions: Dry mouth, blurring of vision, thirst, dizziness, drowsiness, confusion, nervousness, restlessness, nausea, vomiting, diarrhea, double vision, blurring of vision, tingling, heaviness, weakness of hands, tightening of chest, difficulty in urination, constipation, nasal stuffiness, fluttering of heart, headache, insomnia, hives, rash, increased sensitivity to sunlight, low blood pressure, heartburn.

AMCILL® (Parke-Davis and Company)

Generic Name: Ampicillin trihydrate

Dosage Form	Strength	Route
Capsule	250 mg	Oral
	500 mg	Oral
Chewable tablet	125 mg	Oral
Liquid	125 mg/5 ml	Oral
	250 mg/5 ml	Oral
Pediatric drops (liquid)	100 mg/1 ml	Oral

When Prescribed: Amcill is a synthetic penicillin that is effective in a wide variety of infections.

Precautions and Warnings: Amcill should not be taken by people who are allergic to penicillin. The use of any penicillin should be discontinued and your physician notified if any of the side effects or reactions listed below appear.

Side Effects and Adverse Reactions: Nausea, vomiting, chest or stomach pains, diarrhea, blackening of tongue, skin rash, hives, chills, fever, swelling, pain in joints, fainting, super-infection by nonsusceptible organisms, anemia, bruising, indigestion, darkening of the urine.

AMITRIPTYLINE HCl: The generic name for a drug produced by numerous companies, also marketed as:
ELAVIL® Merck Sharp & Dohme

Dosage Form	Strength	Route
Tablet	10 mg	Oral
	25 mg	Oral
	50 mg	Oral
	75 mg	Oral
	100 mg	Oral
	150 mg	Oral

When Prescribed: Amitriptyline hydrochloride is prescribed for relief of symptoms of mental depression or mental depression accompanied by anxiety.

Precautions and Warnings: This drug may impair mental and/or physical abilities required for performance of hazardous tasks, such as operating machinery or driving a motor vehicle. It is not recommended for use by children under 12. Amitriptyline hydrochloride may enhance the response to alcohol and other depressants, such as tranquilizers, sleeping pills, and sedatives. The safe use of amitriptyline hydrochloride in pregnancy has not been established.

Side Effects and Adverse Reactions: Decrease in blood pressure, rapid heart rate, irregular heartbeat upon rising from lying or sitting, stroke, confused state, disturbed concentration, disorientation, delusions, hallucinations, excitement, anxiety, restlessness, insomnia, nightmares, numbness, tingling, loss of balance, tremors, seizures, ringing in ears, dry mouth, blurred vision, constipation, urinary retention, swelling of face and tongue, anemia, nausea, vomiting, heartburn, loss of appetite, diarrhea, swollen glands, black tongue.

AMOXICILLIN The generic name for a drug produced by numerous companies in various forms and strengths. Also marketed as:
AMOXIL® Beecham;
LAROTID® Roche;
POLYMOX® Bristol;
TRIMOX® Squibb;
UTIMOX® Parke Davis
WYMOX® Wyeth.

Generic Name: Amoxicillin

Dosage Form	Strength	Route
Capsule	250 mg	Oral
	500 mg	Oral
Liquid	125 mg/5 ml	Oral
	250 mg/5 ml	Oral

When Prescribed: Amoxicillin is a synthetic penicillin that is prescribed for a wide variety of infections.

Precautions and Warnings: Amoxicillin should not be taken by people who are allergic to penicillin. The use of any penicillin should be discontinued and your physician notified if any of the side effects or reactions listed below appear.

Side Effects and Adverse Reactions: Nausea, vomiting, chest or stomach pains, diarrhea, skin rash, hives, chills, fever, swelling, pain in joints, fainting, superinfection by nonsusceptible organisms, anemia, bruising, indigestion, difficulty in breathing, wheezing.

AMOXIL® (Beecham Laboratories)

Generic Name: Amoxicillin

Dosage Form	Strength	Route
Capsule	250 mg	Oral
	500 mg	Oral
Liquid	125 mg/5 ml	Oral
	250 mg/5 ml	Oral
Liquid (pediatric drops)	50 mg/ml	Oral

When Prescribed: Amoxil is a synthetic penicillin that is prescribed for a wide variety of infections.

Precautions and Warnings: Amoxil should not be taken by people who are allergic to penicillin. The use of any penicillin should be discontinued and your physician notified if any of the side effects or reactions listed below appear.

Side Effects and Adverse Reactions: Nausea, vomiting, chest or stomach pains, diarrhea, skin rash, hives, chills, fever, swelling, pains in joints, fainting, superinfection by nonsusceptible organisms, anemia, bruising, indigestion.

AMPICILLIN
The generic name for a drug produced by numerous companies in various forms and strengths. Also marketed as: AMCILL®, Parke-Davis; OMNIPEN®, Wyeth; PEN-A®, Pfizer; PENBRITEN®, Ayerst; POLYCILLIN®, Bristol.

Generic Name: Ampicillin trihydrate

Dosage Form	Strength	Route
Capsule	250 mg	Oral
	500 mg	Oral
Suspension (liquid)	125 mg/5 cc	Oral
	250 mg/5 cc	Oral

When Prescribed: Ampicillin is a synthetic penicillin that is effective in a wide variety of infections.

Precautions and Warnings: Ampicillin should not be taken by people who are allergic to penicillin. The use of any penicillin should be discontinued and your physician notified if any of the side effects or reactions listed below appear.

Side Effects and Adverse Reactions: Nausea, vomiting, chest or stomach pains, diarrhea, blackening of tongue, skin rash, hives, chills, fever, swelling, pain in joints, fainting, super-infection by nonsusceptible organisms, anemia, bruising, indigestion.

ANAPROX® (Syntex Laboratories, Inc.)

Generic Name: Naproxen sodium

Dosage Form	Strength	Route
Tablet	275 mg	Oral

When Prescribed: Anaprox is prescribed for the relief of mild to moderate pain. It is also prescribed for painful menstruation and to reduce inflammation in joints or other body parts.

Precautions and Warnings: The safe use of this drug during pregnancy has not been established. This drug should not be taken by nursing mothers.

Side Effects and Adverse Reactions: Constipation, heartburn, abdominal pain, nausea, indigestion, diarrhea, stomach pain, headache, dizziness, drowsiness, lightheadedness, vertigo, itching, skin eruptions, bruising, sweating, ringing in the ears, hearing disturbances, visual disturbances, swelling, breathing difficulties, heart flutters, thirst, blood in urine, yellowing of the skin, chills and fever, blood in vomit, dark vomit, blood in the stool, black tarry stool, rash, menstrual disorders, muscle pain, weakness, loss of hair, inability to concentrate, depression, malaise, dream abnormalities.

ANSAID® (Upjohn)

Generic Name: Flurbiprofen

Dosage Form	Strength	Route
Tablets	50 mg	Oral
	100 mg	Oral

When Prescribed: Ansaid is prescribed for the treatment of rheumatoid arthritis and osteoarthritis.

Precautions and Warnings: Ansaid should not be taken by people who have previously had allergic reactions to it or who have reacted with allergic symptoms like asthma or rash to aspirin or to other nonsterodial anti-inflammatory drugs. Gastrointestinal ulceration, bleeding and perforation may occur at any time. Ansaid should be used with caution in patients with kidney or liver disorders, heart problems, and problems of fluid retention.

Side Effects and Adverse Reactions: Indigestion, diarrhea, stomach pain, nausea, constipation, intestinal bleeding, perforation and ulceration, gas, liver abnormalities, vomiting, headache, nervousness, anxiety, insomnia, tremors, nasal inflammation, rash, dizziness, changes in vision, symptoms of urinary tract infection, weight changes.

ANSPOR® (Smith Kline & French)

Generic Name: Cephradine

Dosage Form	Strength	Route
Capsule	250 mg	Oral
	500 mg	Oral
Suspension	125 mg/5 ml	Oral
	250 mg/5 ml	Oral

When Prescribed: Anspor is an antibiotic prescribed for a variety of infections including those of the respiratory tract, ear, bone, skin, and urogenital tract.

Precautions and Warnings: Allergic reactions to Anspor can occur. People who are allergic to penicillin are often allergic to Anspor. This drug should be used in pregnancy only if clearly needed. Caution should be exercised when Anspor is administered to a nursing mother. Safety and effectiveness for infants under 9 months of age have not been established.

Side Effects and Adverse Reactions: Diarrhea, vomiting, nausea, abdominal pain, heartburn, difficulty in breathing, pain in joints, headache, rash, itching, superinfections by nonsusceptible organisms.

ANTIVERT® (Roerig)

Generic Name: Meclizine HCl

Dosage Form	strength	Route
Tablet	12.5 mg	Oral
	25 mg	Oral
Tablet (chewable)	25 mg	Oral

When Prescribed: Antivert is an antihistamine which has been shown to be effective in the management of nausea, vomiting, and dizziness associated with motion sickness. It is possibly effective, though not proved, in management of dizziness associated with diseases of the vestibular (balance) system.

Precautions and Warnings: Antivert is not recommended during pregnancy or for women who may become pregnant while taking the drug, nor is it recommended for preadolescent children. Because drowsiness may occur on occasion, patients should not drive cars or operate dangerous machinery.

Side Effects and Adverse Reactions: Drowsiness, dry mouth and, on rare occasions, blurred vision.

ANUSOL-HC® (Parke-Davis and Company)

Generic Name: Hydrocortisone acetate, bismuth subgallate, bismuth resorcin compound, benzyl benzoate, Peruvian balsam, zinc oxide

Dosage Form	Strength	Route
Suppository	Available in one strength only	Rectal
Cream	Available in one strength only	Rectal

When Prescribed: Anusol-HC is prescribed for the relief of pain and discomfort of hemorrhoids and other disorders of the rectal area.

Precautions and Warnings: The safe use of topical steroids during pregnancy has not been established. Anusol-HC should not be used on extensive areas or for prolonged periods of time in pregnant women.

Side Effects and Adverse Reactions: Local irritation.

APRESOLINE® (Ciba Pharmaceutical Company)

Generic Name: Hydralazine hydrochloride

Dosage Form	Strength	Route
Tablet	10 mg	Oral
	25 mg	Oral
	50 mg	Oral
	100 mg	Oral

When Prescribed: Apresoline is prescribed to reduce blood pressure in patients with high blood pressure.

Precautions and Warnings: Apresoline is a potent drug. Patients using this drug should be closely monitored by their physician. Not recommended during pregnancy.

Side Effects and Adverse Reactions: Headache, heart flutters and rapid heart rate, loss of appetite, nausea, vomiting, diarrhea, chest pains, nasal congestion, flushing, watery eyes, eye irritation, pain, numbness, or tingling in extremities, swelling, dizziness, tremors, muscle cramps, depression, disorientation, anxiety, rash, itching, fever, chills, pain in joints, constipation, difficulty in urination, breathing difficulties.

ARISTOCORT® (Lederle Laboratories)

Generic Name: Triamcinolone

Dosage Form	Strength	Route
Tablet	1 mg	Oral
	2 mg	Oral
	4 mg	Oral
	8 mg	Oral
Syrup	2 mg/15 ml	Oral
Cream	0.025%	Local (apply directly to affected area)
	0.1%	Topical
	0.5%	Topical
Ointment	0.1%	Topical
	0.5%	Topical

When Prescribed: Aristocort (oral) is prescribed for the treatment of different diseases such as hormonal deficiencies, rheumatic disorders, some dermatological problems, allergic reactions, respiratory disorders, abnormalities of blood, certain types of cancer, and gastrointestinal disorders. Aristocort (local) is prescribed for the relief of inflammatory conditions and itching of the skin.

Precautions and Warnings: Aristocort should be used with great caution by pregnant women and nursing mothers. Average and large doses of this drug and other hydrocortisones can cause elevation of blood pressure, salt and water retention, and increase in excretion of potassium. While on this drug, patients should not be vaccinated. Growth and development of infants and children on prolonged corticosteroid therapy should be carefully observed. When using this medicine locally, patients should be advised not to use this medication for any disorder other than that for which it was prescribed. The treated skin area should

ARTANE® (Lederle Laboratories)

Generic Name: Trihexyphenidyl HCl

Dosage Form	Strength	Route
Tablet	2 mg	Oral
	5 mg	Oral
Liquid	2 mg/5 ml	Oral
Capsule (Time Release)	5 mg	Oral

When Prescribed: Artane is prescribed to treat tremors and shaking in patients with Parkinson's disease and certain other nervous system disorders. Artane may also be prescribed to control tremors caused by other drugs.

Precautions and Warnings: Artane therapy is usually prolonged. Frequent physical and eye examinations are necessary.

Side Effects and Adverse Reactions: Dryness of mouth, blurring of vision, dizziness, nausea, nervousness, skin rash, delusions, hallucinations, mental confusion, vomiting, agitation, constipation, drowsiness, urinary difficulties, rapid heartbeat, weakness, headache.

Aristocort-(Continued)

not be bandaged or otherwise covered or wrapped so as to be occlusive unless directed by the physician. Parents of pediatric patients should be advised not to use tight-fitting diapers or plastic pants on a child being treated in a diaper area, as these garments may constitute occlusive dressings.

Side Effects and Adverse Reactions: If patient is taking Aristocort orally, the following are possible side effects and adverse reactions: sodium and fluid retention, congestive heart failure in some

ASENDIN® (Lederle Laboratories)

Generic Name: Amoxapine

Dosage Form	Strength	Route
Tablet	50 mg	Oral
	100 mg	
	150 mg	

When Prescribed: Asendin is prescribed for the relief of symptoms of depression and anxiety.

Precautions and Warnings: Asendin should not be taken with alcohol, sedatives, sleeping pills, or tranquilizers unless directed by your physician. The safe use of this drug in pregnancy has not been established. If drowsiness occurs you should not drive or operate dangerous machinery. Asendin should not be taken by children under the age of 16.

Side Effects and Adverse Reactions: Drowsiness, dry mouth, constipation, visual difficulties, anxiety, insomnia, restlessness, nervousness, heart flutters, tremors, confusion, excitement, nightmares, loss of balance, skin rash, swelling, nausea, dizziness, headache, fatigue, weakness, excessive appetite, increased perspiration, urinary difficulties, fainting, rapid heartbeat, fever, itching, increased sensitivity to sunlight, tingling of skin, unusual sensation in hands or feet, ringing in the ears, disorientation, abnormal movements, seizures, mental disorders, numbness, heartburn, nausea, vomiting, gas, abdominal pain, peculiar taste, diarrhea, change in sex drive, impotence, menstrual problems, breast enlargement, abnormal breast secretions, watery eyes, testicular swelling, loss of appetite, stroke.

ATARAX® (Roerig)

Generic Name: Hydroxyzine HCl, alcohol (liquid only)

Dosage Form	Strength	Route
Tablet	10 mg	Oral
	25 mg	Oral
	50 mg	Oral
	100 mg	Oral
Liquid	Available in one strength only	Oral

When Prescribed: Atarax is prescribed for a wide variety of conditions in which anxiety, tension, and emotional stress are apparent. It is effective in controlling vomiting in stressful situations and for the control of itching in allergic conditions.

Precautions and Warnings: Atarax should not be taken with alcohol, sedatives, sleeping pills or tranquilizers unless specifically directed by your physician. If drowsiness occurs you should not drive or operate dangerous machinery. Atarax should not be taken by nursing mothers or used in early stages of pregnancy.

Side Effects and Adverse Reactions: Drowsiness, dryness of mouth, tremors, convulsions.

Aristocort -(Continued)

patients, decrease in potassium level, increase in blood pressure, muscle weakness, headache, convulsion, vertigo, menstrual irregularities, suppression of growth in children, glaucoma, inflammation of pancreas, peptic ulcer. If a patient is using Aristocort locally, possible side effects and adverse reactions are: burning, itching, irritation, dryness, allergic inflammation of skin, secondary infection.

26

ATIVAN® (Wyeth Laboratories)

Generic Name: Lorazepam

Dosage Form	Strength	Route
Tablet	0.5 mg	Oral
	1.0 mg	Oral
	2.0 mg	Oral

When Prescribed: Ativan is prescribed for relief of the anxiety, tension, agitation, irritability, and insomnia associated with certain emotional or physical disorders.

Precautions and Warnings: This drug should not be taken with sedatives, sleeping pills, or alcohol. Patients who use Ativan should not drive or operate dangerous machinery. Abrupt cessation of this drug after prolonged use may cause withdrawal symptoms. Ativan should not be used by children under 12, by pregnant woman in the first three months of pregnancy, or by nursing mothers.

Side Effects and Adverse Reactions: Sedation, dizziness, weakness, unsteadiness, disorientation, depression, nausea, changes in appetite, headache, sleep disturbance, agitation, skin problems, visual problems, gastrointestinal upset.

ATROVENT® (Boehringer Ingelheim)

Generic Name: Ipratropium Bromide

Dosage Form	Strength	Route
Inhalation Aerosol	14 gm	Oral

When Prescribed: Atrovent is an inhalation aerosol prescribed for the treatment of chronic bronchitis and emphysema.

Precautions and Warnings: Atrovent should not be used by patients allergic to atropine or its derivatives. Atrovent should not be used in acute episodes of bronchospasms where rapid response is needed. It should be used with caution in people with glaucoma, enlarged prostate, and bladder obstruction. To be effective Atrovent must be used consistently throughout the treatment as prescribed. Atrovent should be taken with caution by nursing mothers and pregnant women.

Side Effects and Adverse Reactions: Heart palpitations, nervousness, dizziness, headache, rash, nausea, vomiting, tremor, blurred vision, dry mouth, irritation from aerosol, cough, worsened symptoms.

AUGMENTIN® (Beecham Laboratories)

Generic Name: Amoxicillin, clavulanate potassium

Dosage Form	Strength	Route
Suspension	125 mg	Oral
	250 mg	Oral
Tablet	250 mg	Oral
	500 mg	Oral
	125 mg	Chewable Oral
	250 mg	Chewable Oral

When Prescribed: Augmentin is a combination of amoxicillin and clavulanate potassium. Unlike amoxicillin, this product cannot be destroyed by certain enzymes (lactamase), due to the presence of clavulanate potassium. It is prescribed for a wide variety of infections. It is a synthetic penicillin.

Precautions and Warning: 2 tablets of Augmentin 250 mg should not be used as a substitute for 1 tablet of 500 mg. The drug should not be taken by a person who is allergic to ampicillin. The use of any penicillin, including Augmentin, should be discontinued if any of the following occur.

Side Effects and Adverse Reactions: Nausea, vomiting, chest or stomach pain, diarrhea, skin rash, hives, chills, fever, swelling, pain in joints, fainting, superinfection by nonsusceptible organisms, anemia, bruising, indigestion.

AURALGAN® OTIC SOLUTION
(Ayerst Laboratories)

Generic Name: Antipyrine, benzocaine, glycerin dehydrated, oxyquinoline sulfate

Dosage Form	Strength	Route
Liquid	Available in one strength only	Otic (ear) drops

When Prescribed: Auralgan is prescribed for the relief of pain and the reduction of inflammation in middle-ear infections. It is often used in conjunction with antibiotics. Auralgan is also used to facilitate the removal of ear wax.

Precautions and Warnings: Should not be used by individuals who are sensitive to benzocaine.

Side Effects and Adverse Reactions: No adverse reactions to properly administered Auralgan have been reported.

AVC® CREAM (Merrell-National Laboratories)

Generic Name: Sulfanilamide, aminacrine hydrochloride, allantoin

Dosage Form	Strength	Route
Cream	4-oz. tube	Intravaginal
Suppository	16/box	Intravaginal

When Prescribed: AVC Cream is prescribed for the relief of symptoms caused by infections of the vagina. Symptomatic improvements usually occur in a few days, but treatment is normally continued through one complete menstrual cycle.

Precautions and Warnings: AVC Cream should not be used by patients overly sensitive to sulfonamides, or if any of the adverse reactions listed below occur.

Side Effects and Adverse Reactions: Local discomfort, burning sensation, superinfection by nonsusceptible organisms.

AXID® (Lilly)

Generic Name: Nizatidine

Dosage Form	Strength	Route
Capsule	150 mg	Oral
	300 mg	Oral

When Prescribed: Axid is prescribed for up to 8 weeks in the treatment of duodenal ulcer, with most ulcers healing within 4 weeks.

Precautions and Warnings: Patients with known hypersensitivity to Axid and its components should not take the drug. Relief of symptoms does not rule out cancer. Pregnant women and nursing mothers should use this drug with caution. The safe and effective use of this drug in children have not been established.

Side Effects and Adverse Reactions: Elevated liver enzymes, sweating, itching, rash, fever, nausea.

AZO GANTRISIN® (Roche Laboratories)

Generic Name: Sulfisoxazole, phenazopyridine hydrochloride

Dosage Form	Strength	Route
Tablet	Available in one strength only	Oral

When Prescribed: Azo Gantrisin is prescribed for urinary tract infections, primarily of the kidney and bladder, where pain is a complicating factor and when no urinary obstruction is present.

Precautions and Warnings: Azo Gantrisin is usually not prescribed for children under 12 or for pregnant women at term or nursing mothers. Treatment with Azo Gantrisin should not exceed 2 days. It should not be taken by people sensitive to sulfa drugs and should be taken with adequate fluid intake. The red-orange color of urine after taking this medication is normal.

Side Effects and Adverse Reactions: Sore throat, fever, skin eruptions, skin peeling, hives, itching, nausea, vomiting, abdominal pain, diarrhea, frequent urination, lack of urination, superinfection by nonsusceptible organisms.

BACTRIM® DS (Roche Laboratories)

Generic Name: Trimethoprim, sulfamethoxazole

Dosage Form	Strength	Route
Tablet	Double strength	Oral
Tablet	Regular strength	Oral
Liquid	Available in one strength only	Oral
Pediatric liquid	Available in one strength only	Oral

When Prescribed: Bactrim DS is a combination of drugs prescribed for the treatment of certain infections.

Precautions and Warnings: Bactrim DS is not recommended during pregnancy or for nursing mothers. If any of the side effects or adverse reactions listed below appear, consult your physician.

Side Effects and Adverse Reactions: Rash, sore throat, stomach upset, nausea, vomiting, abdominal pains, diarrhea, yellowing of skin, headache, body aches, depression, convulsions, hallucinations, ringing in the ears, dizziness, loss of balance, insomnia, apathy, fatigue, weakness, nervousness, fever, chills, urinary difficulties.

BACTROBAN® (Beecham Laboratories)

Generic Name: Mupirocin

Dosage Form	Strength	Route
Ointment	2%	Skin

When Prescribed: Bactroban is prescribed to treat impetigo.

Precautions and Warnings: Bactroban should not be used in the eyes. If sensitivity or irritation occurs discontinue use. Avoid the use of Bactroban in pregnant women and nursing mothers.

Side Effects and Adverse Reactions: Burning, stinging, pain, itching, rash, nausea, dry skin, tenderness, redness of the skin, swelling at site of infection or on contact with skin.

BECONASE® (Glaxo Inc.)

Generic Name: Beclomethasone dipropionate

Dosage Form	Strength	Route
Inhaler	Available in one strength only	Nasal Inhalation

When Prescribed: Beconase nasal inhaler is prescribed for relief of symptoms of nasal mucous membrane inflammation which responds poorly to conventional treatment.

Precautions and Warnings: Use of Beconase nasal inhaler should not be continued beyond 3 weeks in the absence of significant symptomatic improvement. Beconase nasal inhaler should not be used in the presence of untreated localized infection involving the nasal mucosa. Patients should use Beconase nasal inhaler at regular intervals, since its effectiveness depends on its regular use. Its use should be avoided by pregnant women and nursing mothers. Safety and effectiveness for children under 12 have not been established.

Side Effects and Adverse Reactions: Irritation and burning of nasal mucosa, sneezing attacks, local infection of the nose.

BEEPEN-VK® (Beecham Laboratories)

Generic Name: Penicillin V Potassium

Dosage Form	Strength	Route
Tablet	125 mg	Oral
	250 mg	Oral
	500 mg	Oral
Liquid	125 mg/5 ml	Oral
	250 mg/5 ml	Oral

When Prescribed: Beepen-VK is a form of penicillin which is prescribed for the treatment of mild to moderately severe infections.

Precautions and Warnings: Penicillin should be used during pregnancy only if clearly needed. Penicillin should be used in nursing mothers with caution. The use of any penicillin should be discontinued and a physician consulted if any of the symptoms listed below appear.

Side Effects and Adverse Reactions: Nausea, vomiting, chest or stomach pains, diarrhea, changes in color/texture of oral membranes, skin rash, hives, chills, fever, swelling, pain in joints, fainting, superinfection by nonsusceptible organisms.

BENTYL® (Lakeside Pharmaceuticals)

Generic Name: Dicyclomine hydrochloride

Dosage Form	Strength	Route
Capsule	10 mg	Oral
	20 mg	Oral
Tablet	Available in one strength only	Oral
Syrup	Available in one strength only	Oral

When Prescribed: Bentyl is prescribed for the treatment of peptic ulcer. It acts by reducing muscle spasm in the gastrointestinal tract. Bentyl may also be useful in other gastrointestinal disorders. The syrup is often prescribed for the treatment of colic in infants.

Precautions and Warnings: If this drug produces drowsiness or blurred vision, you should not drive or operate dangerous machinery. This drug may decrease sweating, which can lead to heat prostration in hot environments.

Side Effects and Adverse Reactions: Dry mouth, urinary difficulties, blurred, vision, rapid heartbeat, heart flutters, visual disturbances, loss of taste, headache, nervousness, drowsiness, weakness, dizziness, insomnia, nausea, vomiting, impotence, suppression of lactation in nursing mothers, constipation, bloated feeling, rash, mental confusion or excitement (especially in older persons), decreased sweating, muscle or skeletal pain.

BETAPEN-VK® (Bristol)

Generic Name: Penicillin V Potassium

Dosage Form	Strength	Route
Tablets	250 mg	Oral
	500 mg	Oral
Oral	125 mg	Oral
Solution	250 mg	Oral

When Prescribed: Betapen-VK is a form of penicillin that is prescribed for the treatment of mild to moderately severe infections.

Precautions and Warnings: Penicillin should be used during pregnancy only if clearly needed, and should be used in nursing mother's with caution. The use of any penicillin should be discontinued and a physician consulted if any of the symptoms listed below appear.

Side Effects and Adverse Reactions: Nausea, vomiting, chest or stomach pains, diarrhea, changes in color/texture of oral membranes, skin rash, hives, chills, fever, swelling, pain in joints, fainting, superinfection.

BETOPTIC™ (Alcon Laboratories, Inc.)

Generic Name: Betaxolol hydrochloride

Dosage Form	Strength	Route
Ophthalmic Solution (eye drop)	Available in one strength only	Eye Drop

When Prescribed: Betoptic is prescribed to lower elevated pressure in the eyes that results from various disorders, including glaucoma.

Precautions and Warnings: Caution should be exercised when Betoptic is used by patients with cardiac failure or lung disease. In pregnancy, it should be used only if clearly needed. This drug is not recommended for use by children.

Side Effects and Adverse Reactions: Eye irritation, rash, itching, reduction in heart rate, insomnia, depressive neurosis.

BLEPHAMIDE® (Allergan Pharmaceuticals, Inc.)

Generic Name: Sulfacetamide sodium, prednisolone acetate

Dosage Form	Strength	Route
Solution (eye drop)	Available in one strength only	Eye Drop

When Prescribed: Blephamide is a combination of antiinfective and steroid. It is prescribed for inflammatory ocular (eye) conditions associated with infection.

Precautions and Warnings: If inflammation or pain persists longer than 48 hours or becomes aggravated, patient should be advised to discontinue the medication and consult physician. To prevent contamination, care should be taken to avoid touching dropper tip to eyelid or any other surface. Blephamide should be used during pregnancy only if clearly needed. Caution should be exercised when Blephamide is administered to a nursing mother. Safety and effectiveness for children below the age of 6 has not been established.

Side Effects and Adverse Reactions: Prolonged use of Blephamide may result in glaucoma with damage to optic nerve; development of secondary infections; delayed wound healing; stinging, burning, and irritation of the eyes.

BLEPH-10® (Allergan Pharmaceuticals, Inc.)

Generic Name: Sulfacetamide sodium

Dosage Form	Strength	Route
Ophthalmic Solution (eye drop)	Available in one strength only	Eye Drop

When Prescribed: Bleph-10 is prescribed for treatment of a number of different eye infections.

Precautions and Warnings: Bleph-10 should not be used by people who are hypersensitive to sulfa drugs. This drug should be stored in a cool place. Upon long standing, the solution will darken in color and should be discarded.

Side Effects and Adverse Reactions: Transient stinging or burning of the eyes.

BRETHINE® (Geigy Pharmaceuticals)

Generic Name: Terbutaline sulfate

Dosage Form	Strength	Route
Tablet	5.0 mg	Oral
	2.5 mg	Oral

When Prescribed: Brethine is prescribed for aiding breathing in patients with asthma, bronchitis, or emphysema.

Precautions and Warnings: This drug should not be used by children under 12 years old.

Side Effects and Adverse Reactions: Nervousness, tremors, headache, rapid heartbeat, heart flutters, drowsiness, nausea, vomiting, sweating, muscle cramps.

BUMEX® (Roche Laboratories)

Generic Name: Bumetanide

Dosage Form	Strength	Route
Tablet	0.5 mg	Oral
	1 mg	Oral

When Prescribed: Bumex is a potent drug that helps the body pass excess water and salt. It is prescribed to treat heart disease, kidney disease, and high blood pressure.

Precautions and Warnings: This drug may cause the loss of potassium from your body. Your doctor may tell you to add special foods to your diet that contain potassium. If a patient is taking Bumex once a day, he is advised to take the drug in the morning so he does not have to get up to urinate during the night. If a patient is allergic to sulfonamides, he may show hypersensitivity to Bumex.

Side Effects and Adverse Reactions: Muscle cramps, electrocardiogram changes, weakness, hives, abdominal pain, arthritic pain, rash, and vomiting.

BUSPAR® (Mead Johnson Pharmaceuticals)

Generic Name: Buspirone Hydrochloride

Dosage Form	Strength	Route
Tablet	5 mg	Oral
	10 mg	Oral

When Prescribed: BuSpar is prescribed for relief of anxiety. Unrelated to sedative drugs, it has shown no evidence of being habit forming.

Precautions and Warnings: BuSpar should not be given to patients hypersensitive to buspirone hydrochloride; used with monoamine oxidase inhibitor, or taken by patients with kidney or liver disease. Since BuSpar may cause drowsiness, do not drive a car or operate machinery. Avoid use of alcohol while on BuSpar therapy. Patients who have been using a CNS depressant may experience withdrawal symptoms. Inform your physician of any medication you are taking, of alcohol consumption, pregnancy and/or breast feeding. The safe and effective use of BuSpar has not been determined in people under 18 years of age.

Side Effects and Adverse Reactions: Dizziness, headache, nervousness, lightheadedness, excitement, insomnia, fatigue, confusion, depression, blurred vision, dry mouth, nausea, diarrhea, constipation, vomiting, aches and pains, numbness, tremors, skin rash, nonspecific chest pain.

BUTAZOLIDIN® (Geigy Pharmaceuticals)

Generic Name: Phenylbutazone

Dosage Form	Strength	Route
Tablet	Available in one strength only	Oral
Capsule		Oral

When Prescribed: Butazolidin is a potent drug prescribed for the relief of pain and inflammation of gout, various forms of arthritis, and other disorders of muscle and bone characterized by pain and inflammation.

Precautions and Warnings: Butazolidin is not considered a simple pain reliever and is never prescribed casually. A patient using this drug should be examined often by his/her physician. Adverse reactions can occur rapidly; therefore the patient should immediately report anything abnormal to his physician. Patients should not drive or operate machinery. Should be taken immediately before or after meals or with milk to minimize gastric irritation.

Note: Rarely used in children under 14 years and in senile patients.

Side Effects and Adverse Reactions: Fever, sore throat, sores in the mouth, indigestion, heartburn, slow-healing cuts, blood which does not clot, easy bruising, dark or bloody stools, significant weight gain, water retention with swelling, stomach or intestinal cramps or pain, nausea, vomiting, diarrhea, bloating, swollen glands, hepatitis, purple spots on skin, itching, general skin eruptions, hives, pains in joints, fever, rash, blood in the urine, frequent urination, lack of urination, kidney stones, painful urination, high blood pressure, pain in the eyes, blurred vision, loss of hearing, increase

BUTISOL SODIUM® (McNeil Laboratories, Inc.)

Generic Name: Sodium butabarbital

Dosage Form	Strength	Route
Tablet	15 mg	Oral
	30 mg	Oral
	50 mg	Oral
	100 mg	Oral
Capsule	15 mg	Oral
	30 mg	Oral
	50 mg	Oral
	100 mg	Oral
Elixir	30 mg/5 cc	Oral

When Prescribed: Butisol Sodium is a barbiturate prescribed as a sedative or a sleeping pill in patients where weaker medications are not deemed effective.

Precautions and Warnings: This drug should not be taken with other sedatives or sleeping pills, or with alcohol or relaxants. Patients using this drug should not drive or operate machinery. Patients using any type of barbiturates for prolonged periods should seek the help of a physician when attempting to discontinue use. Abrupt cessation may be hazardous.

Side Effects and Adverse Reactions: Butisol Sodium may be habit forming. Individuals may develop a psychological dependence on this drug. People who have overused this drug may develop a physical dependence that will result in withdrawal symptoms including convulsions. Adverse reactions include hangover, drowsiness, lethargy, headache, skin eruptions, nausea, vomiting, hives.

Butazolidin-(Continued)

in size of thyroid (in neck), general agitation, confusion, lethargy, salivary gland enlargement, headache, drowsiness, tremors, numbness, weakness, ringing in ears.

CALAN® (Searle and Company)

Generic Name: Verapamil hydrochloride

Dosage Form	Strength	Route
Tablet	80 mg	Oral
	120 mg	Oral

When Prescribed: Calan is prescribed to help prevent attacks of angina that often occur in patients with heart disorders.

Precautions and Warnings: Patients taking Calan should not take any other prescription or nonprescription drugs without informing the physician. In pregnancy, it should be used only when it is clearly needed. It should not be used by nursing mothers.

Side Effects and Adverse Reactions: Hypotension (decrease in blood pressure), pulmonary edema, dizziness, fatigue, headache, constipation, nausea.

CAPOTEN® (E. R. Squibb and Sons, Inc.)

Generic Name: Captopril

Dosage Form	Strength	Route
Tablet	12.5 mg	Oral
	25 mg	Oral
	50 mg	Oral
	100 mg	Oral

When Prescribed: Capoten is prescribed for high blood pressure in patients who have normal kidney function.

Precautions and Warnings: Capoten is a potent drug, so therapy should be started under medical supervision.

Side Effects and Adverse Reactions: Anemia, loss of protein in the urine, hypotension, skin rashes, loss of taste, abdominal pain, vomiting, diarrhea, cough.

CAPOZIDE® (Squibb)

Generic Name: Captopril-Hydrochlorothiazide

Dosage Form	Strength	Route
Tablet	25/15 mg	Oral
	25/25 mg	Oral
	50/15 mg	Oral
	50/25 mg	Oral

When Prescribed: Capozide is prescribed to lower blood pressure.

Precautions and Warnings: In patients with kidney and vascular disease Capozide should be reserved for those who have developed unacceptable side effects on other medication. Swelling of the face, lips, mucous membrane and extremities may occur. If swelling involves the tongue, glottis or larynx, emergency therapy should be immediately initiated. Lowered white blood cell production. Pregnant women and nursing mothers should use Capozide with great caution. This is a potent drug. Close monitoring by your physician is required.

Side Effects and Adverse Reactions: Kidney problems, urinary frequency, anemia, blood clotting, rash, fever, low blood pressure, heart flutters, chest pain, angina, heart attack, reversible taste impairment, cardiac arrest, anemia, hepatitis, confusion, depression, bronchospasms, blurred vision, impotence, nausea, vomiting, diarrhea, cramping, anorexia, jaundice, constipation, hyperglycemia, muscle spasms, weakness, dizziness.

CARAFATE® (Marion Laboratories, Inc.)

Generic Name: Sucralfate

Dosage Form	Strength	Route
Tablet	1 gm	Oral

When Prescribed: Carafate is prescribed for short-term (up to 8 weeks) treatment of duodenal ulcers.

Precautions and Warnings: This drug should be used in pregnancy only when it is clearly needed. Safety and effectiveness for children have not been established.

Side Effects and Adverse Reactions: Constipation, diarrhea, nausea, gastric discomfort, indigestion, dry mouth, rash, back pain, dizziness, sleepiness, vertigo.

CARDIZEM® (Marion Laboratories)

Generic Name: Diltiazem hydrochloride

Dosage Form	Strength	Route
Tablet	30 mg	Oral
	60 mg	Oral

When Prescribed: Cardizem is prescribed to help prevent attacks of angina that often occur in patients with heart disorders.

Precautions and Warnings: Cardizem should not be used by pregnant women, nursing mothers, or children. Cardizem should be used with caution in some heart conditions such as heart failure.

Side Effects and Adverse Reactions: Headache, edema, nausea, dizziness, rash, flushing, hypotension, palpitations, nervousness, insomnia, hallucinations, constipation, dyspepsia, diarrhea, vomiting.

CARDIZEM SR® (Marion)

Generic Name: Diltiazem Hydrochloride

Dosage Form	Strength	Route
Sustained	60 mg	Oral
Release	90 mg	Oral
Capsules	120 mg	Oral

When Prescribed: Cardizem SR is prescribed for the treatment of high blood pressure alone, or in combination with other antihypertensive drugs such as diuretics.

Precautions and Warnings: Cardizem SR is a potent drug. The side effects should be thoroughly discussed with your physician, and Cardizem SR should be used only under close supervision of your physician. The safe use of this drug in pregnancy has not been established. It should not be taken by nursing mothers.

Side Effects and Adverse Reactions: Angina, irregular heartbeat, congestive heart failure, rapid heartbeat, amnesia, depression, gait abnormality, hallucinations, nervousness, personality change, numbness of extremities, tremor, abnormal dreams, liver disease, anorexia, diarrhea, vomiting, weight increase, thirst, rash, dry mouth, impotence, eye irritation, hyperglycemia, sexual difficulties, nasal congestion.

CATAPRES® (Boehringer Ingelheim Ltd.)

Generic Name: Clonidine hydrochloride

Dosage Form	Strength	Route
Tablet	0.1 mg	Oral
	0.2 mg	Oral
	0.3 mg	Oral

When Prescribed: Catapres is prescribed for the treatment of high blood pressure. Catapres is mild to moderate in potency and is often prescribed with other drugs to reduce high blood pressure.

Precautions and Warnings: If drowsiness occurs, you should not drive or operate dangerous machinery. Catapres therapy should not be discontinued without consulting your physician. This drug may enhance the depressive effects of alcohol, sleeping pills, tranquilizers, and sedatives.

Side Effects and Adverse Reactions: Dry mouth, drowsiness, sedation, constipation, dizziness, headache, fatigue, loss of appetite, depression, nausea, vomiting, weight gain, enlargement of breasts, pains in hands or feet, nightmares, insomnia, nervousness, restlessness, anxiety, rash, hives, itching, thinning of hair, impotence, difficulties in urination, dryness of eyes or nose.

CECLOR® (Eli Lilly and Co.)

Generic Name: Cefaclor

Dosage Form	Strength	Route
Liquid	125 mg/5 ml	Oral
	250 mg/5 ml	
Capsule	250 mg	Oral
	500 mg	

When Prescribed: Ceclor is prescribed for a variety of infections, including those of the ear, the respiratory tract, the skin, and urinary tract infections.

Precautions and Warnings: The safe use of this drug in pregnant women and infants less than 1 month of age has not been established. It also may cause allergic reactions in people allergic to penicillins.

Side Effects and Adverse Reactions: Diarrhea, nausea, vomiting, hives, itching, rash, pain in joints, fever, vaginal irritation, superinfection by nonsusceptible organisms.

CENTRAX® (Parke-Davis and Company)

Generic Name: Prazepam

Dosage Form	Strength	Route
Capsule	5 mg	Oral
	10 mg	
Tablet	10 mg	Oral

When Prescribed: Centrax is prescribed for the relief of anxiety in the management of anxiety disorders.

Precautions and Warnings: Patients taking Centrax should not drive or operate dangerous machinery. This drug should not be combined with alcohol, sleeping pills, tranquilizers, or sedatives. Withdrawal from Centrax, especially after prolonged use, can cause adverse reactions.

Side Effects and Adverse Reactions: Fatigue, dizziness, weakness, drowsiness, lightheadedness, lack of coordination, headache, confusion, tremor, abnormal dreams, slurred speech, heart flutters, stimulation, dry mouth, sweating, gastrointestinal disturbances, itching, rashes, swelling of feet, pain in joints, problems in the urinary or genital area, blurred vision, fainting, increase in weight.

CHLORDIAZEPOXIDE

The generic name of a drug produced by numerous companies in various forms and strengths. Also marketed as:
SK-LYGEN®, Smith Kline and French;
LIBRIUM®, Roche;
LIBRATABS®, Roche.

Dosage Form	Strength	Route
Capsule	5 mg	Oral
	10 mg	Oral
	25 mg	Oral
Tablet	5 mg	Oral
	10 mg	Oral
	25 mg	Oral

When Prescribed: For a variety of emotional disorders, including anxiety, tension, and withdrawal symptoms of acute alcoholism. It is also prescribed to relieve the apprehension and anxiety associated with surgery and hospitalization.

Precautions and Warnings: Should not be combined with alcohol, sedatives, tranquilizers, or sleeping pills. Persons using this drug should not drive or operate machinery. Physical and/or psychological dependence can occur with overuse. The use of this drug by pregnant women should almost always be avoided.

Side Effects and Adverse Reactions: Drowsiness, loss of balance, confusion, fainting, skin disorders, swelling, menstrual irregularities, nausea, constipation, altered sex drive, fainting, personality changes.

CIPRO® (Miles Pharmaceutical)

Generic Name: Ciprofloxacin

Dosage Form	Strength	Route
Tablets	250 mg	Oral
	500 mg	Oral
	750 mg	Oral

When Prescribed: Cipro, an antibacterial agent, is prescribed for a variety of infections.

Precautions and Warnings: Generally well-tolerated, Cipro should not be used in children, pregnant women, or lactating mothers. Patients with central nervous system disorders should use Cipro with caution. At the first sign of allergy or rash notify your doctor immediately. Because dizziness or lightheadedness may occur, you should not drive cars, operate machinery, or attempt tasks requiring coordination and alertness while taking this drug. Drink plenty of liquids and do not take antacids containing magnesium or aluminum within two hours of your dosage.

Side Effects and Adverse Reactions: Nausea, diarrhea, abdominal pain, headache, restlessness, rash, gastrointestinal bleeding, dizziness, lightheadedness, heart palpitations.

CLEOCIN® HCL CAPSULES (The Upjohn Company)

Generic Name: Clindamycin HCl hydrate

Dosage Form	Strength	Route
Capsule	75 mg	Oral
	150 mg	Oral
Pediatric Granules		Oral solution

When Prescribed: Cleocin is prescribed for treatment of bacterial infections by susceptible organisms including those of the upper respiratory tract (nose, throat), lower respiratory tract (lungs, bronchial tubes), skin and gums.

Precautions and Warnings: Severe abdominal reactions can occur from the use of Cleocin. If any of the side effects or adverse reactions listed below occurs, Cleocin should be discontinued and your physician consulted. Safety for use in pregnancy has not been established.

Side Effects and Adverse Reactions: Abdominal pain, nausea, vomiting, severe diarrhea, rash, hives, fainting, yellowing of skin or eyes, super-infection by nonsusceptible organisms, pain in joints.

CLINORIL® (Merck, Sharp and Dohme)

Generic Name: Sulindac

Dosage Form	Strength	Route
Tablet	150 mg	Oral
	200 mg	Oral

When Prescribed: Clinoril is prescribed for the relief of pain and inflammation from arthritis, bursitis, and other painful disorders of the joints.

Precautions and Warnings: This drug should not be taken by pregnant women or nursing mothers. It is not recommended that Clinoril and aspirin be taken together.

Side Effects and Adverse Reactions: Gastrointestinal pain, indigestion, nausea, vomiting, diarrhea, constipation, gas, loss of appetite, gastrointestinal cramps, rash, itching, ringing in the ears, swelling, dryness of nose or throat, loss of balance, fever, skin rash, chills.

COGENTIN® (Merck, Sharp and Dohme)

Generic Name: Benztropine mesylate

Dosage Form	Strength	Route
Tablet	0.5 mg	Oral
	1.0 mg	Oral
	2.0 mg	Oral

When Prescribed: Cogentin is prescribed to control the abnormal movements and muscle stiffness associated with Parkinson's disease and certain other diseases.

Precautions and Warnings: The safe use of this drug in pregnancy has not been established. Cogentin may impair the mental and/or physical abilities required to drive a car or operate dangerous machinery. Report any gastrointestinal upsets to your physician immediately. This drug may impair your ability to perspire. This could lead to a dangerous elevation in body temperature in hot environments.

Side Effects and Adverse Reactions: Dry mouth, blurred vision, nausea, nervousness, vomiting, constipation, numbness of the fingers, listlessness, depression, skin rash.

COLY-MYCIN® S OTIC (Parke-Davis)

Generic Name: Colistin sulfate, neomycin sulfate, thonzonium bromide, hydrocortisone acetate otic suspension

Dosage Form	Strength	Route
Liquid	Available in one strength only	Otic (ear) drops

When Prescribed: Coly-mycin S Otic eardrops are prescribed for the treatment of bacterial infections of the external ear canal. They may also be prescribed for infections resulting from operations involving the ear.

Precautions and Warnings: Should not be warmed above body temperature in order to ensure full potency.

Side Effects and Adverse Reactions: Sensitization or irritation of skin, superinfection by nonsusceptible organisms.

COMBID® SPANSULES®
(Smith Kline and French Laboratories)

Generic Name: Prochlorperazine maleate, isopropamide iodide

Dosage Form	Strength	Route
Capsule (Time Release)	Available in one strength only	Oral

When Prescribed: Combid is prescribed as therapy for peptic ulcer and various other gastrointestinal disorders. It is intended to reduce the amount of stomach secretion, reduce spasms and movements of the gastrointestinal tract, relieve anxiety, and tension, and control nausea and vomiting.

Precautions and Warnings: Should not be taken with sleeping pills, sedatives, alcohol, or tranquilizers. If drowsiness occurs, patients should not operate motor vehicles or machinery.

Side Effects and Adverse Reactions: Dry mouth; urinary hesitancy and retention; increased heart rate; irregular heartbeat; dilation of the pupils; inability of the eyes to accommodate to light changes; blurred vision; constipation; bloated feeling; difficulty swallowing; fever; nasal congestion; spasms or jerky movements; tremors; involuntary movements of the face, tongue, or jaws; drowsiness, dizziness; convulsions; headache; impotence; altered personality; low blood pressure; fainting; cardiac arrest; anemia and other blood disorders; yellowing of the skin; lactation; development of breasts in males; menstrual irregularities; false positive pregnancy tests; increased sensitivity to sunlight; itching; hives; rash; allergic reactions; swelling; eye disorders.

COMPAZINE® (Smith Kline and French Laboratories)

Generic Name: Prochlorperazine maleate

Dosage Form	Strength	Route
Suppository	2.5 mg	Rectal
	5 mg	Rectal
	25 mg	Rectal
Tablet	5 mg	Oral
	10 mg	Oral
	25 mg	Oral
Capsule (Time Release) (Spansules®)	10 mg	Oral
	15 mg	Oral
	30 mg	Oral
	75 mg	Oral
Syrup	5 mg/5ml	Oral

When Prescribed: Compazine is prescribed for certain psychotic disorders, for moderate to severe anxiety, and control of severe nausea and vomiting.

Precautions and Warnings: Patients using Compazine may have impaired mental and/or physical abilities, especially during the first few days of therapy. Therefore, patients should not undertake potentially dangerous tasks such as driving or operating machinery. Compazine should not be taken with alcohol, tranquilizers, sedatives, or sleeping pills. Compazine is a potent drug which must be used with caution. Patients noticing any unusual symptoms, including those listed below, should consult a physician immediately.

Side Effects and Adverse Reactions: Drowsiness, dizziness, absence of menstruation, skin disorders, low blood pressure, fainting, jerky movements, tremors, agitation, jitteriness, insomnia, muscle spasms, difficulty swallowing, spasms of eye muscles or tongue, difficulty walking, drooling, abnormal un-

CORDRAN® (Dista Products Company)

Generic Name: Flurandrenolide

Dosage Form	Strength	Route
SP Cream®	.05%	Topical (apply
	.025%	directly to
		affected area)
Lotion	.05%	
Ointment	.05%	
	.025%	

When Prescribed: Cordran is a synthetic equivalent of a substance produced in the body. It is a potent agent prescribed to reduce itching, swelling and inflammation in certain skin disorders.

Precautions and Warnings: Cordran should not be used extensively, in large amounts over large areas, or for prolonged periods of time by pregnant patients.

Side Effects and Adverse Reactions: Skin eruptions, burning, dryness, irritated hair follicles, excessive hair growth, loss of pigment, irritation, itching, destruction of skin.

Compazine-(Continued)

controlled facial movements, convulsions, headache, dryness of mouth, nasal congestion, nausea, constipation, intestinal blockage, impotence, cardiac arrest, anemia and other blood disorders, yellowing of skin, lactation, development of breasts in males, false positive pregnancy tests, increased sensitivity to sunlight, itching, hives, rash, allergic reactions, swelling, eye disorders, blurred vision.

CORGARD® (E. R. Squibb & Sons, Inc.)

Generic Name: Nadolol

Dosage Form	Strength	Route
Tablet	40 mg	Oral
	80 mg	
	120 mg	
	160 mg	

When Prescribed: Corgard is prescribed for long-term management in patients with angina pectoris and is also prescribed to control high blood pressure of patients with hypertension.

Precautions and Warnings: Patients should not discontinue this drug without first consulting their physician. The safety and efficiency of Corgard for children has not been established.

Side Effects and Adverse Reactions: Slow heartbeat, cold extremities, dizziness, fatigue, abnormal skin sensation, sedation, change in behavior, difficulty breathing, nausea, diarrhea, abdominal discomfort, constipation, vomiting, indigestion, loss of appetite, bloating, gas, rash, itching, headache, dry mouth, eyes or skin, decreased sexual drive, impotence, facial swelling, weight gain, slurred speech, cough, nasal stuffiness, sweating, ringing in the ears, blurred vision, depression, loss of hair, disorientation, memory loss, fever, aches, sore throat.

CORTICAINE® (Glaxo Inc.)

Generic Name: Hydrocortisone acetate, dibucaine. Suppository contains hydrocortisone acetate only

Dosage Form	Strength	Route
Cream	Available in one strength only	Topical (apply directly to affected area)
Suppository	Available in one strength only	Intrarectal

When Prescribed: Hydrocortisone acetate (one of the ingredients of Corticaine) is a corticosteroid that reduces swelling and inflammation. The suppository helps relieve symptoms of internal hemorrhoids.

Precautions and Warnings: Corticaine should not be used by patients with tuberculosis or viral or fungal infections. Avoid use of cream in eyes. Do not apply on large areas for prolonged periods of time or use occlusive dressings. Safe and effective use by children has not been established for this product. The recommended duration of treatment for the cream is 2 weeks only.

Side Effects and Adverse Reactions: Burning, itching, irritation, dryness, decrease in pigmentation, allergic reactions, secondary infection.

CORTISPORIN® OTIC DROPS
(Burroughs Wellcome Company)

Generic Name: Polymyxin B sulfate, neomycin sulfate, hydrocortisone

Dosage Form	Strength	Route
Liquid	Available in one strength only	Otic (ear) drops

When Prescribed: Cortisporin Otic ear drops are prescribed for the treatment of bacterial infections of the external ear canal. They may also be prescribed for infections resulting from operations involving the ear.

Precautions and Warnings: To ensure full potency, drops should not be warmed above body temperature. Shake well before using.

Side Effects and Adverse Reactions: Sensitization or irritation of skin, superinfection by nonsusceptible organisms.

COUMADIN® (Endo Laboratories, Inc.)

Generic Name: Crystalline sodium warfarin

Dosage Form	Strength	Route
Tablet	2 mg	Oral
	2.5 mg	Oral
	5 mg	Oral
	7.5 mg	Oral
	10 mg	Oral
	25 mg	Oral

When Prescribed: Coumadin is prescribed for the prevention of blood clots in the veins, certain heart conditions that may lead to clots and clots in the lungs. This drug may also be prescribed for patients who have suffered mild strokes. The aim of Coumadin therapy is to impede the clotting mechanism of the blood, while avoiding spontaneous bleeding.

Precautions and Warnings: Should be taken under strict supervision where the clotting time of the blood is determined periodically. Should not be taken if any of the symptoms listed below appear. Coumadin taken with other drugs can lead to serious interactions. Notify your physician of all prescription and nonprescription drugs which you use. Should not be taken during pregnancy or by nursing mothers.

Side Effects and Adverse Reactions: Major or minor bleeding from any tissue or organ, loss of hair, hives, skin infections, fever, nausea, diarrhea, skin damage due to reduced blood supply, abdominal cramping.

CYCLOCORT® (Lederle Laboratories)

Generic Name: Amcinonide

Dosage Form	Strength	Route
Cream	0.1%	Topical (apply directly to affected area)
Ointment	0.1%	

When Prescribed: Cyclocort is prescribed for relief of inflammation and itching associated with skin disorders.

Precautions and Warnings: Cyclocort should not be used in the eyes. The treated area should not be bandaged or otherwise covered or wrapped by occlusive dressings. This drug should not be used extensively by pregnant women in large amounts or for prolonged periods of time. Prolonged use of Cyclocort by children may interfere with their growth and development.

Side Effects and Adverse Reactions: Burning, itching, irritation, dryness, loss of pigmentation, skin damage, secondary infection.

DALMANE® (Roche Laboratories)

Generic Name: Flurazepam hydrochloride

Dosage Form	Strength	Route
Capsule	15 mg	Oral
	30 mg	Oral

When Prescribed: Dalmane is a sleep-inducing agent useful in all types of insomnia characterized by difficulty in falling asleep, frequent nocturnal awakenings, and/or early morning awakening.

Precautions and Warnings: This drug is not recommended for use by persons under 15 years of age. Patients should not combine Dalmane with alcohol, tranquilizers, sedatives, or other sleeping pills. Patients should not drive or operate heavy machinery after taking this drug. The use of Dalmane during pregnancy should almost always be avoided.

Side Effects and Adverse Reactions: Dizziness, drowsiness, lightheadedness, staggering, loss of balance, falling, severe sedation, lethargy, disorientation, coma, headache, heartburn, upset stomach, nausea, vomiting, diarrhea, constipation, gastrointestinal pain, nervousness, talkativeness, apprehension, irritability, weakness, fluttering of the heart, chest pains, body and joint pains, urinary-genital complaints, sweating, flushing, blurred vision, burning eyes, fainting, low blood pressure, shortness of breath, itching, skin rash, dry mouth, bitter taste, excessive salivation, loss of appetite, euphoria, depression, slurred speech, confusion, restlessness, hallucinations, excitement, stimulation, hyperactivity.

DARVOCET-N® (Eli Lilly and Co.)

Generic Name: Propoxyphene napsylate with acetaminophen

Dosage Form	Strength	Route
Tablet	50	Oral
	100	Oral

When Prescribed: Darvocet-N is prescribed for the relief of mild to moderate pain, either when pain is present alone or when it is accompanied by fever. Darvocet-N contains a nonaspirin pain reliever and fever reducer that is well tolerated by people who are sensitive to aspirin.

Precautions and Warnings: Darvocet-N can cause a psychological and/or physical dependence and withdrawal symptoms. This preparation should not be ingested before undertaking potentially dangerous tasks such as driving or operating machinery, nor should it be taken with alcohol, sedatives, tranquilizers or sleeping pills. The safe use of this drug during pregnancy has not been established.

Side Effects and Adverse Reactions: Dizziness, drowsiness, nausea, vomiting, constipation, abdominal pains, skin rashes, light-headedness, headache, weakness, euphoria, uneasiness, minor visual disturbances.

DARVON® (Eli Lilly and Company)

Generic Name: Propoxyphene hydrochloride

Dosage Form	Strength	Route
Capsule	32 mg	Oral
	65 mg	Oral

When Prescribed: Darvon is prescribed for the relief of mild to moderate pain of any nature. If pain can be controlled with Darvon, it is preferred over stronger narcotic drugs.

Precautions and Warnings: Darvon has potential for abuse and dependency. This drug should not be taken with alcohol, tranquilizers, sedatives, sleeping pills or other central nervous system depressants. The safe use of this drug during pregnancy has not been established. Darvon is not recommended for children. If drowsiness occurs, you should not drive or operate dangerous machinery.

Side Effects and Adverse Reactions: Dizziness, sedation, nausea, vomiting, constipation, abdominal pain, skin rashes, lightheadedness, headache, weakness, euphoria, uneasiness, minor visual disturbances.

DARVON® COMPOUND (Eli Lilly and Company)

Generic Name: Propoxyphene hydrochloride plus aspirin, phenacetin and caffeine

Dosage Form	Strength	Route
Capsule	32 mg	Oral
	65 mg	Oral

When Prescribed: Darvon Compound is prescribed for the relief of mild to moderate pain of any nature. If pain can be controlled with Darvon, it is preferred over stronger narcotic drugs.

Precautions and Warnings: Darvon Compound should not be taken before undertaking potentially dangerous tasks such as driving or operating machinery. Should not be taken with alcohol, sedatives, tranquilizers or sleeping pills. Darvon Compound can produce drug dependence characterized by psychological dependence and, less frequently, physical dependence. The safe use of this drug in pregnancy has not been established. Darvon Compound is not recommended for children.

Side Effects and Adverse Reactions: Dizziness, tiredness, nausea, and vomiting. Other adverse reactions include constipation, abdominal pain, skin rash, lightheadedness, headache, weakness, euphoria, uneasiness, and minor visual disturbances.

DECADRON® (Merck Sharp and Dohme)

Generic Name: Dexamethasone

Dosage Form	Strength	Route
Tablet	.25 mg	Oral
	.50 mg	Oral
	.75 mg	Oral
	1.5 mg	Oral
	4.0 mg	Oral
Elixir	0.5 mg/5 ml	Oral

When Prescribed: Decadron is the man-made equivalent of a substance which is produced naturally in your body by the adrenal glands. The main action of Decadron is to reduce inflammation and swelling. Decadron is prescribed for a variety of reasons including glandular disorders, rheumatic and arthritic disorders, diseases of connective tissues, skin diseases, allergies, eye disorders, respiratory diseases, blood disorders, swelling, meningitis, tuberculosis, gastrointestinal diseases, swelling from dental work.

Precaution and Warnings: Mothers taking Decadron should not nurse. Patients on Decadron therapy should not receive smallpox or other vaccinations. Prolonged use of Decadron may cause psychological and/or physical dependence and subsequent withdrawal symptoms.

Side Effects and Adverse Reactions: Fluid retention, swelling, muscle weakness, ulcer, stomach irritation, slow wound healing, increased sweating, allergic skin reactions, convulsions, dizziness, headache, menstrual irregularities, suppression of growth in children, bulging of the eyes, weight gain, increased appetite, nausea, depressed or "blue" feeling.

DECONAMINE® (Berlex Laboratories, Inc.)

Generic Name: Chlorpheniramine maleate, d-pseudoephedrine hydrochloride (elixir contains alcohol)

Dosage Form	Strength	Route
Tablet	All forms available in one strength only	Oral
SR® Capsules (Time Release)		Oral
Elixir		Oral
Syrup		Oral

When Prescribed: Deconamine is prescribed for the relief of congestion that is often present in colds, hay fever, and allergies.

Precautions and Warnings: Do not take with alcohol, sedatives, tranquilizers, or sleeping pills unless directed by your physician. If drowsiness occurs, you should not drive or operate dangerous machinery. The safe use of this drug in pregnancy has not been established.

Side Effects and Adverse Reactions: Drowsiness, rash, hives, itching, excessive perspiration, increased sensitivity to sunlight, chills, dryness of mouth, nose and throat, headache, heart flutters, rapid heartbeat, sleepiness, dizziness, disturbed coordination, fatigue, confusion, restlessness, excitation, nervousness, tremor, irritability, insomnia, mood changes, abnormal sensations, visual problems, loss of balance, ringing in the ears, hysteria, convulsions, heartburn, loss of appetite, nausea, vomiting, diarrhea, constipation, urinary problems, change in menstrual cycle, thickening of bronchial secretions, tightness of chest, wheezing, nasal stuffiness.

DELTASONE® (The Upjohn Company)

Generic Name: Prednisone

Dosage Form	Strength	Route
Tablet	2.5 mg	Oral
	5.0 mg	Oral
	10 mg	Oral
	20 mg	Oral
	50 mg	Oral

When Prescribed: Deltasone is a hormone which is primarily noted for its potent anti-inflammatory effect. It is prescribed for endocrine disorders, arthritis, collagen disease, skin diseases, allergic reactions, eye diseases, respiratory diseases, blood disorders, cancer of the blood, water retention, and various other diseases.

Precautions and Warnings: Deltasone is a potent drug which should be used only under close supervision of a physician. Patients should not receive smallpox immunization or other inoculations while on Deltasone therapy.

Side Effects and Adverse Reactions: Water retention, heart failure, muscle weakness, loss of muscle, bone fractures, ulcer, abdominal distension, wounds that heal slowly, thin fragile skin, skin eruptions, increased sweating, convulsions, dizziness, headache, menstrual irregularities, masculinization of females, suppression of growth in children, decreased ability to withstand stress, intensification of existing diabetes, cataracts, glaucoma.

DEMEROL® (Winthrop Laboratories)

Generic Name: Meperidene hydrochloride

Dosage Form	Strength	Route
Tablet	50 mg	Oral
	100 mg	Oral
Liquid	50 mg/5 cc	Oral

When Prescribed: Demerol is prescribed for the relief of moderate to severe pain of all types when nonnarcotic pain relievers are not deemed effective.

Precautions and Warnings: Demerol should not be taken before undertaking any potentially hazardous task such as driving or operating machinery. Should not be taken with tranquilizers, pain relievers, sedatives, alcohol or sleeping pills.

Side Effects and Adverse Reactions: Demerol is a narcotic which may be habit forming. Lightheadedness, dizziness, nausea, vomiting and sweating, euphoria, uneasiness, weakness, headache, tremor, uncoordinated muscle movements, hallucinations, disorientation, visual disturbances, dry mouth, constipation, upset stomach, flushing of face, irregular heartbeat, fainting, inability to urinate, itching, hives, skin rash.

DEMULEN® (Searle and Company)

Generic Name: Ethynodiol diacetate with ethinyl estradiol

Dosage Form	Strength	Route
Tablet	Available in one strength only	Oral

When Prescribed: Demulen is an oral contraceptive combining estrogen and progesterone.

Precautions and Warnings: An increased risk of blood clots and other serious disorders has been associated with the use of hormonal contraceptives such as Demulen. Oral contraceptives should be taken only under supervision of a physician. A booklet has been prepared to provide you with additional information. Ask your physician for this booklet. If any of the symptoms listed below appear, discuss continued use of the drug with a physician. Cigarette smoking increases the risk of heart and circulatory trouble as side effects of oral contraceptive use. Women who use oral contraceptives should not smoke.

Side Effects and Adverse Reactions: Nausea, vomiting, stomach cramps, bleeding or spotting at times other than during "period," changes in amount of menstrual flow, absence of menstruation, swelling, abnormal darkening of skin, changes in breasts including tenderness, enlargement, secretion, an increase or decrease in weight, suppression of lactation when taken immediately after childbirth, migraine, rash, rise in blood pressure, mental depression, changes in sex drive, changes in appetite, headache, nervousness, dizziness, fatigue, backache, increase in facial hair, loss of scalp hair, itching.

DESYREL® (Mead Johnson and Company)

Generic Name: Trazodone hydrochloride

Dosage Form	Strength	Route
Tablet	50 mg	Oral
	100 mg	Oral
	150 mg	Oral

When Prescribed: Desyrel is prescribed for the treatment of depression.

Precautions and Warnings: Desyrel should not be taken with alcohol, sleeping pills, tranquilizers, or other depressants without the consent of your physician. The safe use of this drug by people under 18 years of age, pregnant women, and nursing mothers has not been established.

Side Effects and Adverse Reactions: Drowsiness, lightheadedness, dizziness, fatigue, headache, insomnia, nervousness, dry mouth, constipation, blurred vision, painful prolonged penal erection, weight gain, tinnitus, malaise.

53

DEXEDRINE® (Smith Kline and French Laboratories)

Generic Name: Dextroamphetamine sulfate

Dosage Form	Strength	Route
Capsules	5 mg	Oral
	15 mg	Oral
Tablet	5 mg	Oral
Elixir	5mg/5 ml	Oral

When Prescribed: Dexedrine is prescribed for narcolepsy (a sudden uncontrollable disposition to sleep occurring at irregular intervals, with or without predisposing or exciting cause). Dexedrine is also prescribed to help control appetite. It is usually prescribed for a short period of time, during which food intake should also be reduced.

Precautions and Warnings: This drug is related to Amphetamines, a class of drug that has been extensively abused. Dexedrine can produce a psychological dependence. The safe use of this drug in pregnancy has not been established. Dexedrine should not be used by children under 3 years of age to treat narcolepsy. It should not be used by those under the age of 12 for obesity.

Side Effects and Adverse Reactions: Overstimulation, restlessness, dizziness, insomnia, gastrointestinal disturbance, nausea, diarrhea, sweating, headache, dryness of mouth or unpleasant taste, hives, allergic reactions, change in sex drive, psychotic episode, depression following withdrawal of drug.

DIABETA® (Hoechst-Roussel Pharmaceuticals, Inc.)

Generic Name: Glyburide

Dosage Form	Strength	Route
Tablet	1.25 mg	Oral
	2.5 mg	Oral
	5.0 mg	Oral

When Prescribed: Diabeta is prescribed for diabetes (diabetes mellitus) to control the blood sugar levels in addition to diet. It is prescribed after a sufficient trial of dietary therapy has proved unsatisfactory. Diabeta can replace the need for insulin by helping to release the body's own insulin.

Precautions and Warnings: Blood and urine glucose should be monitored periodically while using diabeta. The effect of decreasing blood sugar levels can be potentiated by other drugs. Inform your physician before starting any other medication. Ingestion of alcohol can result in severe vomiting and abdominal cramps. Diabeta should be used during pregnancy only if the potential benefit justifies the potential risk to the fetus. If used during pregnancy Diabeta should be discontinued at least one month prior to the expected delivery date. Safety and effectiveness for children's use of this drug has not been established. Diabeta does not replace the need to restrict diet.

Side Effects and Adverse Reactions: Jaundice, nausea, heartburn, skin rashes, different types of anemia, hypoglycemia (low blood sugar levels), diarrhea, constipation, abdominal pain, gas, itching, weakness, fatigue, loss of balance, drowsiness, dizziness, depression, headache.

DIABINESE® (Pfizer Laboratories Division)

Generic Name: Chlorpropamide

Dosage Form	Strength	Route
Tablet	100 mg	Oral
	250 mg	Oral

When Prescribed: Diabinese is an oral substance that will reduce sugar levels in the blood of adult patients with mild or moderately severe diabetes (diabetes mellitus) which cannot be controlled by diet alone. It can often replace the need for insulin in these patients and is frequently prescribed in conjunction with other oral blood sugar-reducing agents. It is generally not prescribed for children with diabetes.

Precautions and Warnings: The use of alcohol, sedatives, sleeping pills, certain pain relievers, or tranquilizers with Diabinese may lead to adverse side effects. Your physician should be consulted immediately if any side effect or adverse reaction occurs.

Side Effects and Adverse Reactions: Hives, rash, itching, water retention, yellowing of skin or eyes, dark urine, light-colored stools, low-grade fever, sore throat, diarrhea, anemia, loss of appetite, nausea, vomiting, heartburn, weakness, numbness, increased sensitivity to sunlight. If alcohol is taken during the Diabinese treatment, unusual flushing of skin on the face and neck may occur.

DIAMOX® (Lederle Laboratories)

Generic Name: Acetazolamide

Dosage Form	Strength	Route
Tablet	125 mg	Oral
	250 mg	Oral
Capsule	500 mg	Oral

When Prescribed: Diamox is prescribed for edema (water accumulation), epilepsy, and glaucoma. This drug is an enzyme inhibitor effective in the control of fluid secretion.

Precautions and Warnings: Diamox is not recommended for use during pregnancy.

Side Effects and Adverse Reactions: Fever, rash, kidney stones, abnormal skin sensations, loss of appetite, frequent urination, drowsiness, confusion, rash, paralysis, convulsions.

DIAZEPAM The generic name for a drug produced by numerous companies.

Dosage Form	Strength	Route
Tablet	2 mg	Oral
	5 mg	Oral
	10 mg	Oral

When Prescribed: Diazepam is prescribed for a wide variety of problems to provide relief from tension and anxiety. It is used in a wide variety of physical and/or psychological disorders. It is often prescribed along with other drugs for the relief of muscular or skeletal disorders or for the prevention of convulsions. It is helpful in preventing reactions during withdrawal from alcohol.

Precautions and Warnings: Patients taking this drug should not drive or operate machinery. Diazepam should not be taken with alcohol, sedatives, tranquilizers, or sleeping pills. A physical and/or psychological dependence on Diazepam can occur. The use of Diazepam during pregnancy should almost always be avoided.

Side Effects and Adverse Reactions: Drowsiness, fatigue, loss of balance, confusion, constipation, depression, double vision, aches in joints, fainting, frequent urination, yellowing of skin or eyes, changes in sex drive, nausea, changes in salivation, skin rash, slurred speech, tremors, lack of urination, dizziness, blurred vision, anxiety, hallucinations, muscle spasticity, insomnia, rage, sleep disturbances.

DICLOXACILLIN The generic name for a drug produced by numerous companies in different strengths. Also marketed as: DYNAPEN® Bristol; PATHOCIL® Wyeth; DYCILL® Beecham.

Dosage Form	Strength	Route
Capsule	125 mg	Oral
	250 mg	Oral
	500 mg	Oral
Suspension	62.5 mg/5 ml	Oral

When Prescribed: Dicloxacillin is an antibiotic prescribed for a variety of infections.

Precautions and Warnings: This drug should not be taken if the patient has ever had an allergic reaction to any form of penicillin. Patient should take the entire course of therapy prescribed, even if fever and other symptoms have stopped. Discard any liquid form of Dicloxacillin after 7 days if stored at room temperature or after 14 days if refrigerated.

Side Effects and Adverse Reactions: Nausea, vomiting, epigastric discomfort, flatulence, loose stools, skin rash, skin eruptions, hives.

DIDREX® (The Upjohn Company)

Generic Name: Benzphetamine hydrochloride

Dosage Form	Strength	Route
Tablet	25 mg	Oral
	50 mg	

When Prescribed: Didrex is prescribed to help control appetite. It is usually prescribed for a short period of time during which food intake should also be reduced.

Precautions and Warnings: This drug is related to amphetamines, a class of drugs that have been extensively abused. Didrex can produce a psychological dependence. The safe use of this drug in pregnancy has not been established. Didrex should not be used by children under 12 years of age.

Side Effects and Adverse Reactions: Overstimulation, restlessness, dizziness, insomnia, gastrointestinal disturbances, nausea, diarrhea, heart flutters, rapid heartbeat, tremor, sweating, headache, dryness of the mouth or unpleasant taste, hives, allergic reactions involving the skin, changes in sex drive, psychotic episodes, depression following withdrawal of drug.

DIGOXIN The generic name for a drug produced by numerous companies in various forms and strengths.

Generic Name: Digoxin

Dosage Form	Strength	Route
Tablet	.125 mg	Oral
	.25 mg	
	.5 mg	

When Prescribed: Digoxin is a drug which increases the strength of the contractions of the heart. It is prescribed for patients with various forms of heart disease. It may also be used to control an irregular heartbeat.

Precautions and Warnings: Digoxin is a potent drug which can cause serious side effects, particularly if taken in excess. Digoxin should be taken only under the close supervision of a physician to whom any side effects or adverse reactions should be reported.

Side Effects and Adverse Reactions: Loss of appetite, excessive salivation, nausea, vomiting, diarrhea, lethargy, drowsiness, confusion, visual disturbances, blurred vision, changes in color perception, irregular heartbeat, headache, weakness, apathy.

DILANTIN® KAPSEALS® (Parke, Davis and Company)

Generic Name: Diphenylhydantoin sodium

Dosage Form	Strength	Route
Capsule	30 mg	Oral
(Kapseals®)	100 mg	Oral
Liquid	30 mg/5 ml	Oral
	125 mg/5 ml	Oral
Kapseals® D.A.	100 mg	Oral
Tablet (Infatabs)	50 mg	Oral

When Prescribed: Dilantin Kapseals is prescribed for the control of convulsions in patients with epilepsy or in patients with other types of seizures. It may also be used to control an irregular heartbeat.

Precautions and Warnings: Gum disorders occur frequently when this drug is used. The incidence of such disorders may be reduced by good oral hygiene including gum massage, frequent brushing and appropriate dental care. Should be taken with meals to help prevent gastric irritation.

Side Effects and Adverse Reactions: Abnormal eye movements, loss of balance, slurred speech, confusion, dizziness, insomnia, nervousness, twitching, headache, nausea, vomiting, constipation, fever, rash, anemia, enlargement of lymph glands, diseases of the joints, beard growth, hepatitis.

DILAUDID® (Knoll Pharmaceutical Company)

Generic Name: Hydromorphone hydrochloride

Dosage Form	Strength	Route
Tablet	1 mg	Oral
	2 mg	
	3 mg	
	4 mg	
Suppository	3 mg	Rectal

When Prescribed: Dilaudid is prescribed for the relief of moderate to severe pain.

Precautions and Warnings: Dilaudid is a narcotic pain reliever. A physical and/or psychological dependence can occur, especially after prolonged use. This drug should not be taken with alcohol, sleeping pills, tranquilizers, or sedatives unless directed by your physician. If you become drowsy, you should not drive or operate dangerous machinery. The safe use of this drug in pregnancy has not been established. This drug is not recommended for use in children.

Side Effects and Adverse Reactions: Sedation, drowsiness, mental clouding, lethargy, impairment of physical or mental function, anxiety, fear, mood changes, dizziness, psychic dependence, nausea, vomiting, constipation, urinary problems, depression of breathing.

DIMETANE® COUGH SYRUP-DC
(A. H. Robins Company)

Generic Name: Brompheniramine maleate, phenylpropanolamine hydrochloride, alcohol, codeine phosphate

Dosage Form	Strength	Route
Liquid	Available in one strength only	Oral

When Prescribed: Dimetane-DC is prescribed for the relief of cough and thinning of mucus, and for the relief of symptoms of allergy.

Precautions and Warnings: Not recommended for use during pregnancy. Patients are cautioned against engaging in operations which require alertness. Dimetane-DC contains codeine, which may be habit forming.

Side Effects and Adverse Reactions: Rash, hives, drowsiness, lassitude, nausea, dryness of the mouth, dilation of pupils, excitement, irritability, excessive perspiration, chills, headache, heart flutters, rapid heartbeat, sedation, blurred vision, ringing in ears, double vision, convulsions, dizziness, confusion, nervousness, shaking, insomnia, euphoria, loss of appetite, vomiting, diarrhea, constipation, urinary problems, tightness of chest, wheezing, nasal stuffiness, tingling, heaviness, weakness of hands.

DIPROLENE® (Schering Corporation)

Generic Name: Betamethasone dipropionate

Dosage Form	Strength	Route
Ointment	0.05%	Topical (apply directly to affected area)

When Prescribed: Diprolene is prescribed for the relief of inflammation, swelling, itching, and other problems associated with the skin.

Precautions and Warnings: This preparation is not to be used in the eyes. Diprolene should not be used in large amounts or for prolonged periods of time by pregnant women.

Side Effects and Adverse Reactions: The following local adverse reactions can occur: burning, itching, irritation, dryness, inflammation of hair follicles, hair growth, acnelike eruptions, loss of skin color, reddening of skin, changes in appearance of skin.

DIPROSONE® (Schering Corporation)

Generic Name: Betamethasone dipropionate

Dosage Form	Strength	Route
Aerosol (spray)	0.1%	Topical (apply directly to the skin)
Cream	0.05%	Topical
Lotion	0.05%	Topical
Ointment	0.05%	Topical

When Prescribed: Diprosone in its various forms is prescribed for the relief of inflammation, swelling, itching, and other problems associated with the skin.

Precautions and Warnings: These preparations are not to be used in the eyes. Diprosone should not be used in large amounts or for prolonged periods of time in pregnant women.

Side Effects and Adverse Reactions: The following local adverse reactions can occur: burning, itching, irritation, dryness, inflammation of the hair follicles, hair growth, acnelike eruptions, loss of skin color, reddening of skin, changes in the appearance of the skin.

DIPYRIDAMOLE The generic name of a drug produced by numerous companies.

Dosage Form	Strength	Route
Tablet	25 mg	Oral
	50 mg	Oral
	75 mg	Oral

When Prescribed: Dipyridamole is prescribed for long-term management of attack of angina pectoris which results from heart disease. Dipyridamole is not to be used for pain of an acute anginal attack. Acute anginal attacks are usually treated with nitroglycerin. Dipyridamole works by increasing blood flow in coronary vessels of the heart.

Precautions and Warnings: Angina pectoris results from heart disease which could be fatal. Report any side effects or unusual reactions to your physician at once.

Side Effects and Adverse Reactions: Headache, nausea, flushing, weakness, fainting, gastrointestinal upset, rashes, chest or shoulder pain.

DISALCID® (Riker Laboratories, Inc.)

Generic Name: Salsalate

Dosage Form	Strength	Route
Tablet	500 mg	Oral
	750 mg	Oral
Capsule	500 mg	Oral

When Prescribed: Disalcid is an analgesic prescribed for relief of signs and symptoms of arthritis. It can be given safely to patients who are sensitive to aspirin.

Precautions and Warnings: Disalcid is not recommended for patients suffering from chicken pox, influenza, or flu symptoms. It should not be used with other salicylates. Disalcid should be used with caution in pregnancy. The safe and effective use by children has not been established.

Side Effects and Adverse Reactions: Ringing in the ears, temporary hearing loss, nausea, heartburn, gastric irritation.

DITROPAN® (Marion Laboratories)

Generic Name: Oxybutyrin chloride

Dosage Form	Strength	Route
Tablet	Available in one strength only	Oral

When Prescribed: Ditropan is prescribed for relief of symptoms associated with voiding in patients with bladder abnormality.

Precautions and Warnings: If Ditropan is given to a patient in the presence of high environmental temperature, it can cause fever or heat stroke due to decreased sweating. Ditropan should not be used in pregnancy. Ditropan is not recommended for children under the age of 5. Ditropan should be given with caution to the elderly and all patients with liver or kidney disease.

Side Effects and Adverse Reactions: Dry mouth, decreased sweating, urinary retention, blurred vision, increase in heart rate, drowsiness, dilation of pupils, sleep disturbances, suppression of lactation, nausea, vomiting, constipation, weakness, dizziness.

DOLOBID® (Merck Sharp and Dohme)

Generic Name: Diflunisal

Dosage Form	Strength	Route
Tablet	250 mg	Oral
	500 mg	Oral

When Prescribed: Dolobid is prescribed for acute or long-term treatment of symptoms of arthritis. Dolobid has a lower incidence of adverse gastrointestinal effects than does aspirin. Patients treated with Dolobid also had a lower incidence of hearing loss and ringing in the ears.

Precautions and Warnings: Dolobid should not be used in pregnancy, by nursing mothers, or patients with gastric ulcers. Dolobid should not be used by patients who exhibit bronchospastic reactivity to aspirin.

Side Effects and Adverse Reactions: Nausea, vomiting, dyspepsia, gastrointestinal pain, diarrhea, constipation, flatulence, insomnia, dizziness, rash, headache, fatigue, tiredness.

DONNAGEL®-PG (A. H. Robins Company)

Generic Name: Kaolin, hyoscyamine sulfate, atropine sulfate, hyoscine hydrobromide, alcohol, opium, pectin

Dosage Form	Strength	Route
Liquid	Available in one strength only	Oral

When Prescribed: Donnagel-PG is prescribed for the control of acute, nonspecific diarrhea where milder, nonprescription drugs are not considered effective.

Precautions and Warnings: Donnagel-PG contains opium, which may be habit forming.

Side Effects and Adverse Reactions: Blurring of vision, dry mouth, difficult urination, flushing and dryness of the skin, irregular heartbeat, constipation.

DONNATAL® (A. H. Robins Company)

Generic Name: Hyoscyamine sulfate, atropine sulfate, hyoscine hydrobromide, phenobarbital, alcohol (liquid only)

Dosage Form	Strength	Route
Tablet	Each form is	Oral
Capsule	available in one	Oral
No. 2 Tablets	strength only	Oral
Liquid (Elixir)		Oral
Time Release Tablet		Oral

When Prescribed: Donnatal is prescribed for the treatment of ulcers and other forms of intestinal distress.

Precautions and Warnings: Donnatal contains phenobarbital, which may be habit forming.

Side Effects and Adverse Reactions: Blurred vision, dry mouth, difficult urination, flushing or dryness of the skin.

DOXYCYCLINE The generic name for a drug produced by numerous companies.

Dosage Form	Strength	Route
Capsule	50 mg	Oral
	100 mg	Oral
Tablet	100 mg	Oral

When Prescribed: Doxycycline is derived from tetracycline and is an antibiotic prescribed for a variety of infections.

Precautions and Warnings: Doxycycline should not be taken by people overly sensitive to tetracycline. If any of the side effects listed below occur, consult your physician. This drug should not be taken by pregnant women, infants, or children under 8.

Side Effects and Adverse Reactions: Exaggerated sunburn, superinfection by non-susceptible organisms, loss of appetite, nausea, vomiting, diarrhea, inflammation of the tongue, difficulty swallowing, stomach pains, inflammation of the bowel and genital region, skin rash, hives, swelling, fainting.

DUOFILM® (Stiefel Laboratories)

Generic Name: Salicylic acid, lactic acid

Dosage Form	Strength	Route
Liquid	16.7%	Topical (apply directly to the affected area)

When Prescribed: Duofilm is prescribed for treatment of common warts.

Precautions and Warnings: Duofilm should not be used by diabetics or patients with abnormal blood circulation. Do not use on moles, birthmarks, or unusual warts with hair growing from them. Duofilm should not allowed to contact normal skin surrounding warts. Duofilm is only for external use. Do not permit Duofilm to contact eyes or mucosal membranes. Duofilm is highly flammable and should be kept away from fire or flame.

Side Effects and Adverse Reactions: Localized irritation will occur if Duofilm is applied to normal skin surrounding the wart.

DURICEF® (Mead Johnson Pharmaceutical Division)

Generic Name: Cefadroxil monohydrate

Dosage Form	Strength	Route
Liquid	125 mg/5 ml	Oral
	250 mg/5 ml	
	500 mg/5 ml	
Tablet	1000 mg	Oral
Capsule	500 mg	Oral

When Prescribed: Duricef is an antibiotic prescribed for a variety of infections including those of the urinary tract, the skin, and the nose and throat.

Precautions and Warnings: This drug may cause allergic reactions in people who are allergic to penicillin.

Side Effects and Adverse Reactions: Nausea, diarrhea, urinary difficulties, rash, hives, itching or pain in the genital area, superinfection by nonsusceptible organisms.

E.E.S.® (Abbott Laboratories)

Generic Name: Erythromycin®
ethylsuccinate

Dosage Form	Strength	Route
Chewable tablet	200 mg	Oral
Infants' drops	100 mg/dropper	Oral
Liquid	200 mg/ teaspoon	Oral
	400 mg/ teaspoon	Oral
Granules for suspension	200 mg/ teaspoon (5cc)	Oral
Filmtabs®	400 mg	Oral

When Prescribed: E.E.S. is prescribed for a wide variety of infections. It is often prescribed for infections where penicillin would normally be the drug of choice but the patient has a sensitivity to penicillin.

Precautions and Warnings: E.E.S. is an antibiotic which can cause an allergic reaction. The safety of this drug during pregnancy has not been established.

Side Effects and Adverse Reactions: Abdominal cramping or discomfort, nausea, vomiting, diarrhea, superinfection by nonsusceptible organisms, hives, rash, fainting.

Elavil -(Continued)

swelling of testicles and enlargement of breasts in males, increased breast size and excessive milk flow in females, changes in sex drive, dizziness, weakness, fatigue, headache, considerable weight change, increased perspiration, frequent urination, dilation of pupils, drowsiness, yellowing of skin or eyes, loss of hair. Abrupt cessation after long-term therapy may cause headache, weakness, and fatigue.

ELAVIL® (Merck Sharp and Dohme)

Generic Name: Amitriptyline HCl

Dosage Form	Strength	Route
Tablet	10 mg	Oral
	25 mg	Oral
	50 mg	Oral
	75 mg	Oral
	100 mg	Oral
	150 mg	Oral

When Prescribed: Elavil is prescribed for the relief of symptoms of mental depression or mental depression accompanied by anxiety.

Precautions and Warnings: This drug may impair mental and/or physical abilities required for performance of hazardous tasks such as operating machinery or driving a motor vehicle. It is not recommended for use by children under 12 years of age. Elavil may enhance the response to alcohol and other depressants such as tranquilizers, sleeping pills and sedatives. The safe use of Elavil in pregnancy has not been established.

Side Effects and Adverse Reactions: Decreases in blood pressure, rapid heart rate, irregular heartbeat upon rising from lying or sitting, stroke, confusional states, disturbed concentration, disorientation, delusions, hallucinations, excitement, anxiety, restlessness, insomnia, nightmares, numbness, tingling, incoordination, loss of balance, tremors, seizures, ringing in the ears, dry mouth, blurred vision, discomfort of eyes, constipation, inability to urinate, rash, hives, increased sensitivity of skin to light, swelling of face and tongue, anemia, nausea, vomiting, heartburn, loss of appetite, peculiar tastes, diarrhea, swollen glands, black tongue,

EMPIRIN® with CODEINE (Burroughs Wellcome Company)

Generic Name: Aspirin, codeine

Dosage Form	Strength	Route
Tablet	No. 2	Oral
	No. 3	Oral
	No. 4	Oral

When Prescribed: Empirin with Codeine is prescribed for the relief of mild, moderate, and moderate to severe pain. No. 4 contains the most codeine and is prescribed for moderate to severe pain. Nos. 2 and 3 are prescribed for less severe pain.

Precautions and Warnings: This drug contains codeine which may be habit forming. Should be used with caution when taking nervous system depressants such as tranquilizers, sleeping pills, sedatives, or alcohol. If drowsiness occurs, you should not drive or operate dangerous machinery.

Side Effects and Adverse Reactions: Lightheadedness, dizziness, sedation, nausea, vomiting, mood changes, constipation, itching, headache, loss of balance, ringing in the ears, mental confusion, drowsiness, sweating, thirst, stomach upset, rash.

E-MYCIN® (The Upjohn Company)

Generic Name: Erythromycin

Dosage Form	Strength	Route
Tablet	250 mg	Oral
	333 mg	Oral

When Prescribed: E-Mycin is prescribed for a wide variety of infections. It is often prescribed for infections when penicillin would normally be the drug of choice but the patient has a sensitivity to penicillin.

Precautions and Warnings: E-Mycin is an antibiotic which can cause an allergic reaction in susceptible individuals. The safe use of this drug in pregnancy has not been established.

Side Effects and Adverse Reactions: The most frequent side effects of erythromycin preparations are gastrointestinal, such as abdominal cramping, discomfort, nausea, vomiting, and diarrhea. Other reactions include superinfection by nonsusceptible organisms, hives, rash, and fainting.

ENDURON® (Abbott Laboratories)

Generic Name: Methyclothiazide

Dosage Form	Strength	Route
Tablet	2.5 mg	Oral
	5 mg	Oral

When Prescribed: Enduron is prescribed for treatment of high blood pressure, fluid accumulation due to congestive heart failure, cirrhosis of the liver, kidney disease, and other conditions where water accumulation is a symptom. Enduron helps the kidneys to pass water and salt thereby reducing water retention.

Precautions and Warnings: Enduron is a potent drug that should be used only under close supervision of your physician. This drug should not be taken by nursing mothers.

Side Effects and Adverse Reactions: Dryness of mouth, thirst, weakness, lethargy, drowsiness, restlessness, muscle pains or cramps, muscular fatigue, frequent urination, rapid heartbeat, nausea, vomiting, loss of appetite, gastric upset, gastrointestinal cramps, constipation, dizziness, loss of balance, abnormal skin sensation, headache, rash, hives, skin eruptions, jaundice, yellow appearance of objects, diarrhea, sensitivity to sunlight.

ENTEX® (Norwich-Eaton Pharmaceuticals)

Generic Name: Phenylephrine hydrochloride, phenylpropanolamine hydrochloride, guaifenesin, alcohol (liquid only)

Dosage Form	Strength	Route
Capsule		Oral
	Both forms available in one strength only	
Liquid		Oral

When Prescribed: Entex is prescribed for the relief of symptoms of colds and other respiratory infections and for allergies and ear infections.

Precautions and Warnings: The safe use of Entex in pregnancy has not been established. This drug should not be taken by nursing mothers.

Side Effects and Adverse Reactions: Nervousness, insomnia, restlessness, headache, nausea, stomach irritation, difficulty urinating.

ENTEX LA® (Norwich-Eaton Pharmaceuticals)

Generic Name: Phenylpropanolamine hydrochloride, guaifenesin

Dosage Form	Strength	Route
Tablet	Available in one strength only	Oral

When Prescribed: Entex LA is prescribed for the relief of symptoms of certain respiratory disorders and to help break up mucus that often accompanies the infections.

Precautions and Warnings: The safe use of this drug in pregnancy has not been determined. Entex LA should not be taken by nursing mothers. This drug is not recommended for children under 12 years of age. Do not crush or chew the tablet.

Side Effects and Adverse Reactions: Nervousness, insomnia, restlessness, headache, difficulty in urination.

EQUAGESIC® (Wyeth Laboratories)

Generic Name: Meprobamate, acetylsalicylic acid

Dosage Form	Strength	Route
Tablet	Available in one strength only	Oral

When Prescribed: Equagesic is prescribed for relief of anxiety and tension in patients with mild pain caused by various disease states. It is also used to promote sleep in tense and anxious patients.

Precautions and Warnings: Overuse of this drug can lead to physical and/or psychological dependence. Sudden withdrawal after prolonged and excessive use may cause adverse reactions. Equagesic may impair the mental or physical abilities required for the performance of potentially hazardous tasks such as driving or operating machinery. Should not be taken with alcohol, tranquilizers, sedatives, or sleeping pills. Equagesic is not recommended for pregnant women, nursing mothers, or children under 6.

Side Effects and Adverse Reactions: Drowsiness, loss of balance, dizziness, slurred speech, headache, weakness, tingling, crawling skin, inability of eyes to adapt to changing light, euphoria, stimulation, excitement, nausea, vomiting, diarrhea, irregular heartbeat, fainting, itching, rash, hives, anemia, swelling, fever, chills.

ERYC® (Parke-Davis and Company)

Generic Name: Erythromycin

Dosage Form	Strength	Route
Capsule	250 mg	Oral

When Prescribed: Eryc is prescribed for a wide variety of infections. It is often prescribed for infections when penicillin would normally be the drug of choice but the patient has a sensitivity to it.

Precautions and Warnings: Eryc is an antibiotic which can cause severe allergic reactions. The safety of this drug during pregnancy has not been established.

Side Effects and Adverse Reactions: Abdominal cramping or discomfort, nausea, vomiting, diarrhea, anorexia, liver dysfunction, eczema.

ERYPED® (Abbott Laboratories)

Generic Name: Erythromycin ethylsuccinate

Dosage Form	Strength	Route
Granules for Suspension	500 mg/5 ml (1 teaspoon)	Oral

When Prescribed: Eryped is prescribed for a wide variety of infections. It is often prescribed for infections when penicillin would normally be the drug of choice but the patient has a sensitivity to it.

Precautions and Warnings: Eryped is an antibiotic which can cause an allergic reaction. The safety of this drug during pregnancy has not been established. After constitution, Eryped must be stored below 77° F (25° C) and used within 35 days. Refrigeration is not required.

Side Effects and Adverse Reactions: Abdominal cramping or discomfort, nausea, vomiting, diarrhea, superinfection by nonsusceptible organisms, hives, rash, fainting.

ERY-TAB® (Abbott Laboratories)

Generic Name: Erythromycin

Dosage Form	Strength	Route
Tablet	250 mg	Oral
	333 mg	Oral
	500 mg	Oral

When Prescribed: Ery-Tab is prescribed for a wide variety of infections. It is often prescribed for infections when penicillin would normally be the drug of choice but the patient has a sensitivity to it.

Precautions and Warnings: Ery-Tab is an antibiotic that can cause an allergic reaction in susceptible individuals. The safe use of this drug in pregnancy has not been established.

Side Effects and Adverse Reactions: The most frequent side effects of erythromycin preparations are gastrointestinal—such as abdominal cramping, discomfort, nausea, vomiting, and diarrhea. Other reactions include: superinfection by nonsusceptible organisms, hives, rash, fainting.

ERYTHROCIN® STEARATE (Abbott Laboratories)

Generic Name: Erythromycin stearate

Dosage Form	Strength	Route
Tablet	125 mg	Oral
(Filmtab®)	250 mg	Oral
	500 mg	Oral

When Prescribed: Erythrocin is prescribed for a wide variety of infections. It is often prescribed for infections when penicillin would normally be the drug of choice but the patient has a sensitivity to penicillin.

Precautions and Warnings: Erythrocin is an antibiotic which can cause an allergic reaction in susceptible individuals. Best absorption is on an empty stomach. The safe use of this drug during pregnancy has not been established.

Side Effects and Adverse Reactions: Abdominal cramping, discomfort, nausea, vomiting and diarrhea, superinfection by nonsusceptible organisms, hives, rash, and fainting.

ERYTHROMYCIN

ERYTHROMYCIN The generic name for a drug produced by numerous companies in various forms and strengths. Also marketed as:
E-MYCIN® Upjohn;
ERYTHROCIN® Abbott;
PEDIAMYCIN® Ross;
PFIZER-E® Pfizer.

Generic Name: Erythromycin

Dosage Form	Strength	Route
Tablet	250 mg	Oral
	500 mg	Oral

When Prescribed: Erythromycin is prescribed for a wide variety of infections. It is often prescribed for infections when penicillin would normally be the drug of choice but the patient has a sensitivity to penicillin.

Precautions and Warnings: Erythromycin is an antibiotic which can cause an allergic reaction in susceptible individuals. The safe use of this drug in pregnancy has not been established.

Side Effects and Adverse Reactions: The most frequent side effects of erythromycin preparations are gastrointestinal, such as abdominal cramping, discomfort, nausea, vomiting, and diarrhea. Other reactions include superinfection by nonsusceptible organisms, hives, rash, and fainting.

ESTRADERM ESTRADIOL TRANSDERMAL system®
(CIBA Pharmaceutical)

Generic Name: Estrogen, Estradiol Transdermal System

Dosage Form	Strength	Route
Skin Patch	.05 mg	Skin
	.01 mg	Skin

When Prescribed: Estraderm is prescribed for the relief of many unpleasant symptoms of menopause including hot flashes and night sweats, offering continuous delivery for twice-weekly application.

Precautions and Warnings: Estrogens may increase the risk of cancer of the uterus in postmenopausal women exposed to the drug for more than one year and should not be used during pregnancy. There is no evidence that "natural" estrogens are more or less hazardous than "synthetic" dosages. Estrogens should not be used in women or men with: breast cancer, pregnancy, undiagnosed genital bleeding, or heart disease. A complete family and medical history should be taken and evaluated prior to estrogen therapy. Estrogens may cause fluid retention in patients with a predisposition.

Side Effects and Adverse Reactions: Breakthrough bleeding and other menstrual disorders, enlarged tumors, breast tenderness and enlargement, nausea, vomiting, stomach cramps, bloating, intolerance to contact lenses, headache, dizziness.

FASTIN® (Beecham Laboratories)

Generic Name: Phentermine hydrochloride

Dosage Form	Strength	Route
Capsule	Available in one strength only	Oral

When Prescribed: Fastin is prescribed for a short period of time (usually a few weeks) in conjunction with a diet for the reduction of body weight in people who are overweight and cannot lose weight by diet alone.

Precautions and Warnings: Fastin may interfere with your ability to drive or operate machinery. This drug is related to the class of compounds known as amphetamines and, therefore, has potential for abuse and drug dependency. Fastin should not be used by children under 12.

Side Effects and Adverse Reactions: Heart flutters, excessive stimulation, restlessness, dizziness, insomnia, mood changes, tremor, headache, psychotic behavior, dryness of mouth, unpleasant taste, diarrhea, constipation, rash, changes in sex drive, impotence.

FELDENE® (Pfizer Laboratories Division)

Generic Name: Piroxicam

Dosage Form	Strength	Route
Capsule	10 mg 20 mg	Oral

When Prescribed: Feldene is prescribed to reduce the pain and swelling of osteoarthritis and rheumatoid arthritis.

Precautions and Warnings: This drug is not recommended for use in children, pregnant women, or nursing mothers.

Side Effects and Adverse Reactions: Stomach irritation, loss of appetite, heartburn, nausea, constipation, abdominal discomfort, gas, diarrhea, abdominal pain, indigestion, dizziness, sleepiness, loss of balance, ringing in the ears, headache, depression, swelling, itching, rash, vomiting, blood in vomit, blood in stool, black vomit or stool, dry mouth, sweating, red blotching of skin, bruising, skin problems, swollen eyes, blurred vision, eye irritation, blood in urine, change in weight, insomnia, nervousness, restlessness, heart flutters, breathing difficulties, painful urination.

FIORICET® (Sandoz Pharmaceuticals)

Generic Name: Butalbital, caffeine, acetaminophen

Dosage Form	Strength	Route
Tablet	Available in one strength only	Oral

When Prescribed: Fioricet is a combination of a mild sedative and a pain reducer. It is prescribed for pain of nervous tension or headache, or any pain brought on by tension or anxiety.

Precautions and Warnings: Fioricet contains a barbiturate which may be habit forming. Excessive and prolonged use should be avoided. If drowsiness occurs, you should not drive or operate dangerous machinery. Fioricet should not be given to children under 12.

Side Effects and Adverse Reactions: Drowsiness, nausea, dizziness, rash, lightheadedness, flatulence, mental confusion.

FIORINAL® (Sandoz Pharmaceuticals)

Generic Name: Butalbital, caffeine, aspirin

Dosage Form	Strength	Route
Tablet	Available in one strength only	Oral
Capsule	Available in one strength only	Oral

When Prescribed: Fiorinal is a combination of a mild sedative and a pain reducer. It is prescribed for relief of pain of nervous tension headache or any pain brought on by tension or anxiety. It is also prescribed for reduction of pain and/or fever in conditions such as arthritis, menstrual cramps, the common cold, and dental extractions.

Precautions and Warnings: Fiorinal contains a barbiturate which may be habit forming. Excessive or prolonged use should be avoided. If drowsiness occurs, you should not drive or operate dangerous machinery. Fiorinal should not be used by children under 12.

Side Effects and Adverse Reactions: Drowsiness, nausea, dizziness, rash, lightheadedness, flatulence.

FIORINAL® with CODEINE (Sandoz Pharmaceuticals)

Generic Name: Butalbital, caffeine, aspirin, codeine phosphate

Dosage Form	Strength	Route
Capsule	No. 1	Oral
	No. 2	Oral
	No. 3	Oral

When Prescribed: Fiorinal with Codeine is prescribed for the relief of pain resulting from a variety of conditions. It may also reduce the urge to cough, making it useful for respiratory infections, acute colds, bronchitis, and other conditions in which cough and pain are symptoms.

Precautions and Warnings: Fiorinal may be habit forming. If drowsiness occurs, you should not drive or operate dangerous machinery.

Side Effects and Adverse Reactions: Nausea, vomiting, constipation, dizziness, skin rash, drowsiness, change in pupil size.

FLAGYL® (Searle and Company)

Generic Name: Metronidazole

Dosage Form	Strength	Route
Tablet	250 mg	Oral
	500 mg	Oral

When Prescribed: Flagyl is prescribed for treatment of certain infections (trichomoniasis) of the genital tract in both males and females. It is also prescribed for treatment of dysentery (amebic dysentery) and liver abscess caused by amoebas.

Precautions and Warnings: Alcoholic beverages should not be consumed during Flagyl therapy because abdominal cramps, vomiting, and flushing may occur. This drug is not recommended for use during early pregnancy. Should not be used by nursing mothers.

Side Effects and Adverse Reactions: Nausea, headache, loss of appetite, vomiting, diarrhea, heartburn, cramps, constipation, unpleasant metallic taste, furry tongue, sore throat, dizziness, incoordination, loss of balance, numbness, crawling skin, joint pains, confusion, irritability, depression, insomnia, rash, weakness, hives, dryness of mouth, itching, painful urination, fever, painful sexual intercourse, frequent urination, decreased sex drive, nasal congestion, pus in urine, inflammation of bowel, darkening of urine, superinfection by nonsusceptible organisms.

FLEXERIL® (Merck Sharp and Dohme)

Generic Name: Cyclobenzaprine

Dosage Form	Strength	Route
Tablet	10 mg	Oral

When Prescribed: Flexeril is prescribed along with rest and physical therapy for the relief of muscle spasms or stiffness associated with disorders of the muscles or skeleton. Flexeril is usually only to be taken for a period of two to three weeks.

Precautions and Warnings: Flexeril may impair your physical and/or mental ability to drive or operate machinery. This drug should not be taken by nursing mothers or by children under 15.

Side Effects and Adverse Reactions: Drowsiness, dry mouth, dizziness, increased heart rate, weakness, fatigue, indigestion, nausea, abnormal sensations in skin, unpleasant taste, blurred vision, insomnia, sweating, muscle pains, breathing difficulties, abdominal pain, constipation, coated tongue, tremors, joint pain, euphoria, nervousness, disorientation, confusion, headache, urinary difficulties, loss of coordination, mood depression, hallucinations, rash, swelling of face or tongue, heart flutters, disturbed concentration, delusions, excitement, anxiety, nightmares, seizures, ringing in the ears, eye problems, increased sensitivity to sunlight, vomiting, loss of appetite, upset stomach, swollen glands, black tongue, yellowing of skin, swelling of testicle and development of breasts in males, increase in breast size and secretion in females, changes in sex drive, weight gain or loss, loss of hair.

FML® (Allergan Pharmaceuticals)

Generic Name: Fluorometholone

Dosage Form	Strength	Route
Ophthalmic (eye) Suspension	Available in one strength only	Eye Drops

When Prescribed: FML is prescribed for steroid-responsive inflammatory conditions of the eye.

Precautions and Warnings: Prolonged use of FML may result in glaucoma and optic nerve damage. It should not be used for fungal infections or tuberculosis of the eye. The safety and effectiveness of this product have not been established for children under the age of 2.

Side Effects and Adverse Reactions: Glaucoma, optic nerve damage, visual disturbances, secondary infection, increase in internal pressure in the eye.

FOLIC ACID The generic name for a drug produced by numerous companies.

Dosage Form	Strength	Route
Tablet	1 mg	Oral

When Prescribed: Folic acid is prescribed to treat anemia due to general folic acid deficiency. It is also prescribed for anemias in pregnancy, infancy, and childhood.

Precautions and Warnings: Some of the anemias cannot be treated with folic acid alone, and these conditions may also require vitamin B.

Side Effects and Adverse Reactions: Allergic conditions.

FUROSEMIDE The generic name of a drug produced by numerous companies.

Dosage Form	Strength	Route
Tablet	20 mg	Oral
	40 mg	Oral
	80 mg	Oral

When Prescribed: Furosemide is a potent drug which helps the body pass excess water and salt, causing a prompt and copious flow of urine. It is used in the treatment of heart disease, liver problems, kidney disease, and high blood pressure. It is used where weaker agents are not deemed as effective.

Precautions and Warnings: Furosemide is not recommended for pregnant women, however, it is safe and effective in infants and children when used as directed in the prescribing information. Furosemide should be taken only under the close supervision of your physician.

Side Effects and Adverse Reactions: Abdominal pain or distension, nausea, vomiting, weakness, fatigue, dizziness, lethargy, leg cramps, loss of appetite, mental confusion, hives, itching, skin reactions, numbness, tingling of skin, blurring of vision, diarrhea, anemia, ringing in the ears, deafness, sweet taste, oral or gastric burning, swelling, headache, yellowing of skin or eyes, blood clots, thirst, increased perspiration, urinary frequency.

GANTRISIN® (Roche Laboratories)

Generic Name: Acetyl sulfisoxazole

Dosage Form	Strength	Route
Tablet	Available in one strength only	Oral
Syrup	Available in one strength only	Oral
Pediatric Suspension	Available in one strength only	Oral

When Prescribed: Gantrisin is a sulfonamide, which is an antibacterial agent used to treat urinary tract infections, meningitis, ear infections, and various other infections.

Precautions and Warnings: Gantrisin is usually not prescribed during pregnancy, at term, or during the nursing period. It should be accompanied by adequate fluid intake.

Side Effects and Adverse Reactions: Sore throat, fever, paleness, yellowing of skin or eyes, rash, anemia, skin eruptions, hives, itching, swelling, nausea, vomiting, diarrhea, loss of appetite, dizziness, insomnia, frequent urination, lack of urination, superinfection by nonsusceptible organisms.

GARAMYCIN® CREAM (Schering Corporation)

Generic Name: Gentamicin sulfate

Dosage Form	Strength	Route
Cream	0.1%	Topical (apply directly to affected area)
Ointment	0.1%	Topical

When Prescribed: Garamycin is prescribed for a wide variety of bacterial skin infections. Whether the cream or ointment is prescribed depends on the nature of the infection.

Precautions and Warnings: Garamycin is not effective against fungal infections. Occasionally fungal infections can occur in the same area being treated with Garamycin.

Side Effects and Adverse Reactions: Irritation of skin, itching.

GEOCILLIN® (Roerig)

Generic Name: Carbenicillin indanyl sodium

Dosage Form	Strength	Route
Tablet	382 mg	Oral

When Prescribed: Geocillin is a semi-synthetic penicillin. It is prescribed for treatment of acute and chronic infections of the urinary tract, prostate, skin, and respiratory tract.

Precautions and Warnings: Geocillin should not be used by people who are allergic to penicillin. The use of any penicillin including geocillin should be discontinued and the physician notified if any of the side effects or reactions listed below appear.

Side Effects and Adverse Reactions: Nausea, vomiting, diarrhea, chest or stomach pain, skin rash, blackening of tongue, swelling, pain in joints, superinfections by nonsusceptible organisms, dry mouth, inflammation of vagina.

GLUCOTROL® (Roerig)

Generic Name: Glipizide

Dosage Form	Strength	Route
Tablet	5 mg	Oral
	10 mg	Oral

When Prescribed: Glucotrol is prescribed for diabetes (diabetes mellitus) to control the blood sugar levels in addition to diet. It is prescribed after a sufficient trial of dietary therapy has proved unsatisfactory. Glucotrol can replace the need for insulin by helping to release the body's own insulin.

Precautions and Warnings: Blood and urine glucose should be monitored periodically while using Glucotrol. The effect of decreasing blood sugar levels can be potentiated by other drugs. Inform your physician before starting any other medication. Ingestion of alcohol can result in severe vomiting and abdominal cramps. Glucotrol should be used during pregnancy only if the potential benefit justifies the potential risk to the fetus and should be discontinued at least one month prior to the expected delivery date. Safety and effectiveness for children's use of this drug has not been established. Glucotrol does not replace the need to restrict diet.

Side Effects and Adverse Reactions: Jaundice, nausea, heartburn, skin rashes, different types of anemia, hypoglycemia (low blood sugar levels), diarrhea, constipation, abdominal pain, gas, itching, weakness, fatigue, loss of balance, drowsiness, dizziness, depression, headache.

GYNE-LOTRIMIN® (Schering Corporation)

Generic Name: Clotrimazole

Dosage Form	Strength	Route
Cream	1%	Intravaginal
Vaginal Tablet	100 mg	Intravaginal

When Prescribed: Gyne-Lotrimin is prescribed for certain infections of the vagina commonly known as yeast infections.

Precautions and Warnings: If relief is not evident in seven to fourteen days, see your physician again.

Side Effects and Adverse Reactions: Vaginal burning, irritation, painful urination.

HALCION® (The Upjohn Company)

Generic Name: Triazolam

Dosage Form	Strength	Route
Tablet	0.125 mg	Oral
	0.25 mg	Oral
	0.5 mg	Oral

When Prescribed: Halcion is prescribed for relief of anxiety, tension, and insomnia associated with emotional or physical disorders.

Precautions and Warnings: Halcion can produce physical and/or psychological dependence. Halcion should not be discontinued abruptly after prolonged use. This drug should not be taken with alcohol, tranquilizers, sleeping pills, or sedatives unless directed by your physician. This drug should not be taken by pregnant women, nursing mothers, or children under the age of 18.

Side Effects and Adverse Reactions: Drowsiness, headache, dizziness, nervousness, lightheadedness, coordination disorders, nausea, vomiting, euphoria, tachycardia, memory impairment, cramps/pain, depression, visual disturbances.

HALDOL® (McNeil Laboratories)

Generic Name: Haloperidol

Dosage Form	Strength	Route
Tablet	0.5 mg	Oral
	1.0 mg	Oral
	2.0 mg	Oral
	5.0 mg	Oral
	10 mg	Oral
Liquid	Available in one strength only	Oral

When Prescribed: Haldol is prescribed for the management of certain emotional disorders. It is often prescribed for extremely hyperactive children.

Precautions and Warnings: If drowsiness occurs, you should not drive or operate dangerous machinery. This drug should not be taken with alcohol. Nursing mothers should not use this drug.

Side Effects and Adverse Reactions: Tremors, stiffness, abnormal jerky movements, involuntary movements of tongue, face, mouth, or jaw, insomnia, restlessness, anxiety, mood alterations, agitation, drowsiness, lethargy, headache, confusion, loss of balance, seizures, hallucinations, rapid heartbeat, yellowing of the skin, rash, loss of hair, increased sensitivity to sunlight, changes in sex drive, menstrual disorders, breast enlargement, impotence, loss of appetite, constipation, diarrhea, excessive salivation, nausea, vomiting, indigestion, dry mouth, blurred vision, urinary difficulties, breathing difficulties.

HISMANAL® (Janssen Pharmaceutical)

Generic Name: Astemizole

Dosage Form	Strength	Route
Tablet	10 mg	Oral

When Prescribed: Hismanal is an antihistamine prescribed for the relief of symptoms of seasonal allergies and skin rashes.

Precautions and Warnings: Patients with known allergies to astemizole should not take Hismanal. Patients with asthma and kidney problems should use Hismanal with caution. Risk of harmful outcomes is potentiated in pregnant and nursing mothers.

Side Effects and Adverse Reactions: Drowsiness, headache, fatigue, appetite and weight increase, nervousness, dizziness, nausea, diarrhea, stomach pain, dry mouth, conjunctivitis, pain in the joints.

HYCODAN® (Endo Laboratories, Inc.)

Generic Name: Hydrocodone bitartrate, homatropine methylbromide

Dosage Form	Strength	Route
Tablet	Both forms available in one strength only	Oral
Syrup		Oral

When Prescribed: Hycodan is prescribed for the control of cough.

Precautions and Warnings: Hycodan contains a narcotic that can be habit forming. A physical and/or psychological dependence on this drug can develop with prolonged use. If drowsiness occurs, you should not drive or operate dangerous machinery. Hycodan should not be taken with alcohol, sleeping pills, sedatives or tranquilizers unless specifically directed by your physician.

Side Effects and Adverse Reactions: Sedation, nausea, vomiting, constipation.

HYCOMINE® SYRUP (Endo Laboratories, Inc.)

Generic Name: Hydrocodone bitartrate, phenylpropanolamine hydrochloride

Dosage Form	Strength	Route
Liquid	Available in one strength only	Oral

When Prescribed: Hycomine is prescribed to control cough and provide relief of congestion in the upper respiratory tract due to the common cold and other ailments.

Precautions and Warnings: Hycomine contains a narcotic which may be habit forming. Patients should not drive or operate machinery while taking this medication.

Side Effects and Adverse Reactions: Drowsiness, heart flutters, dizziness, nervousness, gastrointestinal upset.

HYDERGINE® (Sandoz Pharmaceuticals)

Generic Name: Dihydroergocornine mesylate, dihydroergocristine mesylate, dihydroergokryptine mesylate

Dosage Form	Strength	Route
Tablet	0.5 mg	Sublingual
	1.0 mg	(dissolve under tongue)
Tablet	0.5 mg	Oral
	1.0 mg	Oral

When Prescribed: Hydergine is prescribed for elderly patients to help reduce some of the symptoms that can accompany old age such as depression, confusion, unsociability, dizziness; and is used to treat migraine headaches.

Precautions and Warnings: Hydergine should be taken under close supervision of your physician.

Side Effects and Adverse Reactions: Irritation under tongue, transient nausea, stomach upset.

HYDRALAZINE HYDROCHLORIDE

The generic name of a drug produced by numerous companies in different strengths. Also marketed as:
Apresoline® Ciba Pharmaceutical Company.

Dosage Form	Strength	Route
Tablet	10 mg	Oral
	25 mg	Oral
	50 mg	Oral
	100 mg	Oral

When Prescribed: Hydralazine hydrochloride is prescribed to reduce blood pressure in patients with high blood pressure.

Precautions and Warnings: Hydralazine hydrochloride is a potent drug. Patients using this drug should be closely monitored by their physician. Not recommended during pregnancy.

Side Effects and Adverse Reactions: Headache; heart flutters and rapid heart rate; loss of appetite; nausea; vomiting; diarrhea; chest pains; nasal congestion; flushing; watery eye; eye irritation; pain, numbness, or tingling in extremities; swelling; dizziness; tremors; muscle cramps; depression; disorientation; anxiety; rash; itching; fever; chills; pain in joints; constipation; difficulty in urination; breathing difficulties.

HYDROCHLOROTHIAZIDE The generic name for a drug produced by numerous companies in various forms and strengths. Also marketed as: ESIDREX®, Ciba; HYDRODIURIL®, Merck Sharp and Dohme; ORETIC®, Abbott; THIURETIC®, Parke, Davis & Co.

Generic Name: Hydrochlorothiazide

Dosage Form	Strength	Route
Tablet	25 mg	Oral
	50 mg	Oral
	100 mg	Oral

When Prescribed: Hydrochlorothiazide is prescribed for treatment of high blood pressure or for treatment of water accumulation due to congestive heart failure, cirrhosis of the liver, kidney disease, or other conditions in which water retention is a problem. Hydrochlorothiazide helps the kidneys to pass water and salt.

Precautions and Warnings: This is a potent drug. Frequent check-ups by your physician are required during hydrochlorothiazide therapy. This drug should not be taken by nursing mothers.

Side Effects and Adverse Reactions: Dryness of mouth, thirst, weakness, lethargy, drowsiness, restlessness, muscle pains or cramps, muscular fatigue, urinary disturbances, rapid heartbeat, loss of appetite, stomach irritation, nausea, vomiting, stomach cramps, diarrhea, constipation, dizziness, loss of balance, numbness or tingling of skin, headache, yellow appearance of objects, rash, hives, itching.

HYDROCODONE W/APAP® The generic name for a drug produced by numerous companies in various forms and strengths. Also marketed as: Vicodin Knoll: Other producers include: Barr Geneva Rugby

Dosage Form	Strength	Route
Tablet	5/500 mg	Oral

When Prescribed: Hydrocodone W/APAP is prescribed for the relief of moderate to moderately severe pain.

Precautions and Warnings: Hydrocodone W/APAP may be habit forming. This is a potent drug which may impair your mental and/or physical abilities. Patients using this drug should not drive or operate machinery. The safe use of Hydrocodone W/APAP in pregnancy and nursing mothers has not been established. As with all narcotics, use of this drug prior to delivery may depress respiratory function in the newborn. It should be used with caution in the elderly, very sick patients and those with kidney or liver problems.

Side Effects and Adverse Reactions: Lie down when you feel lightheadedness, dizziness, sedation, nausea and vomiting. Dependence, drowsiness, mental fog, anxiety, fear, constipation, respiratory depression.

HYDROCORTISONE CREAM The generic name for a drug produced by numerous companies.

Dosage Form	Strength	Route
Cream	0.5%	Topical (Apply directly to affected area)
	1.0%	
	2.5%	

When Prescribed: Hydrocortisone cream is prescribed for various skin problems characterized by swelling, itching, redness, and pain.

Precautions and Warnings: Use of hydrocortisone cream over large surface areas, over a long time period, and with occlusive dressings should be avoided. It should also be used with great caution by pregnant women, nursing mothers, and children.

Side Effects and Adverse Reactions: Burning, itching, irritation, dryness, decrease in pigmentation, secondary infection.

HYDRODIURIL® (Merck Sharp and Dohme)

Generic Name: Hydrochlorothiazide

Dosage Form	Strength	Route
Tablet	25 mg	Oral
	50 mg	Oral
	100 mg	Oral

When Prescribed: Hydrodiuril helps the body to pass excess water and salt. It is often prescribed in cases of heart disease, liver problems, kidney disease. Hydrodiuril is also prescribed for high blood pressure.

Precautions and Warnings: Mothers should not nurse while taking this drug.

Side Effects and Adverse Reactions: Loss of appetite, stomach irritation, nausea, vomiting, cramps, diarrhea, constipation, dizziness, loss of balance, numbness, pain or tingling in hands, headache, yellow appearance of objects, faintness, rash, hives, fevers, respiratory distress, sensitivity to sunlight, muscle spasms, weakness, restlessness, transient blurred vision.

HYDROXYZINE HYDROCHLORIDE

The generic name of a drug produced by numerous companies in various strengths. Also marketed as:
ATARAX® Roerig;
DURRAX® Durmik;
NEUCALM® Legere.

Dosage Form	Strength	Route
Tablet	10 mg	Oral
	25 mg	Oral
	50 mg	Oral
	100 mg	Oral
Syrup	10 mg/5 ml	Oral

When Prescribed: Prescribed for a wide variety of conditions in which anxiety, tension, and emotional stress are apparent. It is effective in controlling vomiting in stressful situations and for the control of itching in allergic conditions.

Precautions and Warnings: Should not be taken with alcohol, sedatives, sleeping pills, or tranquilizers unless specifically directed by your physician. If drowsiness occurs, you should not drive or operate dangerous machinery. Should not be taken by nursing mothers or used in early stages of pregnancy.

Side Effects and Adverse Reactions: Drowsiness, dryness of mouth, tremors, convulsions.

HYGROTON® (USV Laboratories, Inc.)

Generic Name: Chlorthalidone

Dosage Form	Strength	Route
Tablet	25 mg	Oral
	50 mg	Oral
	100 mg	Oral

When Prescribed: Hygroton helps the body pass excess water and salt and is prescribed for use in management of high blood pressure. It may also be prescribed, along with other drugs, for heart disease, liver problems, kidney disorders and during pregnancy.

Precautions and Warnings: Mothers should not nurse while taking this drug.

Side Effects and Adverse Reactions: Dryness of mouth, thirst, weakness, lethargy, drowsiness, restlessness, muscle pains or cramps, muscle fatigue, low blood pressure, frequent urination, rapid heartbeat, nausea, vomiting, loss of appetite, diarrhea, constipation, yellowing of skin or eyes, gastrointestinal distress, dizziness, numbness, headache, yellow appearance of objects, anemia, rash, hives, increased sensitivity to sunlight, fever, respiratory distress, blurred vision, upset stomach, intestinal cramps, impotence.

HYTONE® (Dermik Laboratories, Inc.)

Generic Name: Hydrocortisone

Dosage Form	Strength	Route
Cream	0.5% 1.0% 2.5%	Topical (apply directly to the affected area)
Ointment	0.5% 1.0%	Topical

When Prescribed: Hytone is prescribed for various skin problems characterized by swelling, itching, reddening, or pain.

Precautions and Warnings: This product should not be used in large amounts or for prolonged periods of time in pregnant women. This drug is not for use in the eyes.

Side Effects and Adverse Reactions: Burning, itching, irritation, dryness, infection of hair follicles, hair growth, acne-like eruptions, loss of skin color, loss of skin, reddening of the skin, abnormal appearance of the skin.

HYTRIN® (Abbott)

Generic Name: Terazosin Hydrochloride

Dosage Form	Strength	Route
Tablet	1 mg	Oral
	2 mg	Oral
	5 mg	Oral
	10 mg	Oral

When Prescribed: Hytrin is prescribed for the treatment of high blood pressure.

Precautions and Warnings: Low blood pressure is associated with the first few doses of Hytrin. Hytrin can cause drowsiness, thus impairing the ability to drive or operate machinery. When symptoms of low blood pressure occur, sit down.

Side Effects and Adverse Reactions: Weakness, tiredness, fatigue, back pain, headache, palpitations, low blood pressure, rapid heartbeat, nausea, swelling, weight gain, painful extremities, depression, dizziness, decreased sex drive, nervousness, indigestion, nasal congestion, sinusitis, blurred vision, impotence.

IBUPROFEN
The generic name for a drug produced by numerous companies in various strengths. Also marketed as:
RUFEN® Boots;
MOTRIN® Upjohn.

Dosage Form	Strength	Route
Tablet	300 mg	Oral
	400 mg	Oral
	600 mg	Oral
	800 mg	Oral

When Prescribed: Ibuprofen is prescribed to relieve pain and inflammation of arthritis. Ibuprofen is as effective as aspirin for long-term management of pain and inflammation but usually is better tolerated in terms of stomach upset and irritation.

Precautions and Warnings: Ingestion of ibuprofen is not recommended during pregnancy or for nursing mothers. The use of aspirin with ibuprofen may reduce the effectiveness of the drug.

Side Effects and Adverse Reactions: Nausea, chest pain, heartburn, diarrhea, constipation or gastric pain, abdominal cramps or pain, vomiting, indigestion, bloating, gas, dizziness, headache, nervousness, rash, ringing in the ears, decreased appetite, depression, insomnia, visual disturbances, nightmares, fever, itching.

ILOSONE® (Dista Products Division of Eli Lilly and Company)

Generic Name: Erythromycin estolate

Dosage Form	Strength	Route
Liquid	125 mg/5 ml	Oral
	250 mg/5 ml	Oral
Capsule	125 mg	Oral
(Pulvules®)	250 mg	Oral
Tablet	500 mg	Oral
Tablets	125 mg	Oral
(chewable)	250 mg	Oral
Drops	100.mg/1 ml	Oral

When Prescribed: Ilosone is prescribed for a wide variety of infections. It is often prescribed for infections where penicillin would normally be the drug of choice but the patient has a sensitivity to penicillin.

Precautions and Warnings: Ilosone is an antibiotic which can cause an allergic reaction in susceptible individuals. Serious liver complications have been reported with Ilosone use. This may be accompanied by a general poor feeling, nausea, vomiting, fever or abdominal distress. Patients experiencing any of these symptoms should contact a physician immediately.

Side Effects and Adverse Reactions: The most frequent side effects of erythromycin preparations are gastrointestinal, such as abdominal cramping, discomfort, nausea, vomiting and diarrhea. Other reactions include superinfection by nonsusceptible organisms, hives, rash, fainting, fever, jaundice.

ILOTYCIN® (Dista Products Companies)

Generic Name: Erythromycin

Dosage Form	Strength	Route
Tablet	250 mg	Oral
Ophthalmic Ointment	5 mg/gm	Eye Ointment

When Prescribed: Ilotycin tablets are prescribed for various kinds of infections. Ilotycin eye ointment is prescribed for eye infections involving the conjunctiva and cornea.

Precautions and Warnings: The use of antimicrobial agents including Ilotycin may be associated with the overgrowth of antibiotic-resistant organisms. Safety of erythromycin has not been established in pregnancy. Erythromycin is an antibiotic which can cause allergic reactions.

Side Effects and Adverse Reactions: Sensitivity reactions when used in the eyes. When used orally, patients may suffer with the following: abdominal cramps, nausea, vomiting, diarrhea, superinfection by nonsusceptible organism, hives, rash, fainting.

IMIPRAMINE HCL: The generic name for a drug produced by numerous companies in different strengths. Also marketed as: JANIMINE FILMTAB® (Abbott); SK-PRAMINE® (Smith Kline and French); TOFRANIL® (Geigy).

Dosage Form	Strength	Route
Tablet	10 mg	Oral
	25 mg	Oral
	50 mg	Oral

When Prescribed: Imipramine HCl is prescribed for the relief of symptoms of depression. It may also be prescribed to control daytime frequency of urination and to control bed-wetting in individuals older than 6.

Precautions and Warnings: This drug can impair mental and/or physical abilities. Alcohol should not be used with this drug. Imipramine HCl can lead to serious and sometimes fatal reactions if taken with certain other drugs. Be sure to inform your physician of all drugs you take. Mothers should not nurse while taking this drug.

Side Effects and Adverse Reactions: Changes in blood pressure, irregular heartbeat, stroke, fainting, confusion, hallucinations, disorientation, delusions, anxiety, restlessness, agitation, insomnia, nightmares, numbness or tingling sensation, incoordination, loss of balance, tremors, ringing in the ears, dry mouth, blurred vision, trouble adapting to changing light, dilation of pupils, constipation, difficulty urinating, allergic skin disorders, anemia, sore throat, nausea, vomiting, heartburn, strange taste, abdominal cramps, black tongue, breast enlargement in males, breast enlargement and lactation in females, change in sexual behavior, swelling of testicles,

IMODIUM® (Ortho Pharmaceutical Corp.)

Generic Name: Loperamide hydrochloride

Dosage Form	Strength	Route
Capsule	2 mg	Oral

When Prescribed: Imodium is prescribed for diarrhea. It is also prescribed to reduce the volume of discharge from surgical openings of the bowel (ileostomies).

Precautions and Warnings: The safe use of Imodium during pregnancy has not been established. This drug should not be taken by nursing mothers or children under 12 years of age.

Side Effects and Adverse Reactions: Abdominal pain, abdominal distension, abdominal discomfort, constipation, dizziness, drowsiness, dry mouth, nausea, vomiting, tiredness, rash.

INDERAL® (Ayerst Laboratories)

Generic Name: Propranolol hydrochloride

Dosage Form	Strength	Route
Tablet	10 mg	Oral
	20 mg	Oral
	40 mg	Oral
	80 mg	Oral

When Prescribed: Inderal is a potent drug which is prescribed for various, often serious, heart conditions such as angina pectoris. It is intended to help the heart beat at a normal rhythm. It is also used to control symptoms of certain tumors of the nervous system, for high blood pressure, and for migraine headache.

Precautions and Warnings: Patients using this drug should be closely monitored, and should not abruptly discontinue the drug after long-term use. If any of the side effects listed below appear, your physician should be contacted immediately.

Side Effects and Adverse Reactions: Slow heartbeat, heart failure, low blood pressure, numbness or tingling of the hands, lightheadedness, insomnia, lassitude, weakness, fatigue, mental depression, visual disturbances, hallucinations, disorientation, memory loss, changes in emotions, nausea, vomiting, heartburn, cramps, diarrhea, constipation, rash, fever, sore throat, respiratory distress, anemia, loss of hair.

Imipramine HCl-(Continued)

yellow skin or eyes, change in weight, perspiration, frequent urination, dizziness, weakness, fatigue, loss of appetite, diarrhea, black tongue, loss of hair.

INDERAL® LA (Ayerst Laboratories)

Generic Name: Propranolol hydrochloride (LA stands for <u>long acting</u>)

Dosage Form	Strength	Route
Capsule	80 mg	Oral
	120 mg	Oral
	160 mg	Oral

When Prescribed: Inderal LA is a potent drug which is prescribed for various, often serious heart conditions, such as angina pectoris. It is intended to help the heart beat at a normal rhythm. It is also used to control high blood pressure and migraine headaches. The only difference between Inderal and Inderal LA is that patients take Inderal LA on a once-daily basis.

Precautions and Warnings: Patients using this drug should be closely monitored and should not discontinue using this drug abruptly after long-term use. If any of the side effects listed below appear, contact your physician. Patients suffering from asthma or any other respiratory problems should inform their physician before starting this drug.

Side Effects and Adverse Reactions: Slow heart rate, decrease in blood pressure, nausea, vomiting, lightheadedness, mental depression, insomnia, abdominal cramping, diarrhea, constipation, bronchospasms.

INDERIDE® (Ayerst Laboratories)

Generic Name: Propranolol hydrochloride, hydrochlorothiazide

Dosage Form	Strength	Route
Tablet	40/25	Oral
	80/25	

When Prescribed: Inderide is prescribed for the management of high blood pressure. It is usually prescribed only after other medications have been ineffective.

Precautions and Warnings: The safe use of this drug in pregnancy has not been established. This drug should not be taken by nursing mothers. Patients using Inderide should be closely monitored, and should not abruptly discontinue the drug after long-term use.

Side Effects and Adverse Reactions: Slow heartbeat, altered sensation in the hands, cold extremities, lightheadedness, mental depression, insomnia, lassitude, weakness, fatigue, visual disturbances, hallucinations, disorientation, memory loss, mood changes, nausea, vomiting, heartburn, abdominal cramping, diarrhea, constipation, sore throat, rash, fever, aches, breathing difficulties, easy bruising, loss of hair, eye irritation, loss of appetite, yellowing of skin, yellow appearance of objects, dizziness, loss of balance, headache, increased sensitivity to sunlight, restlessness, blurred vision.

INDOCIN® (Merck Sharp and Dohme)

Generic Name: Indomethacin, MSD

Dosage Form	Strength	Route
Capsule	25 mg	Oral
	50 mg	Oral
Cap. Sust. Release	75 mg	Oral

When Prescribed: Indocin is a potent drug prescribed for relief of pain and swelling in various forms of arthritis where less potent drugs are not effective.

Precautions and Warnings: Indocin is not a simple pain reliever. It should be taken only under close supervision of your physician. Indocin is usually not prescribed for children under 14, pregnant women or nursing mothers. In patients who chronically use Indocin, periodic eye examinations should be made. Elderly patients are more susceptible to the adverse side reactions. Patients should not drive or operate machinery while taking Indocin. Should be taken with food, immediately after meals or with antacid to minimize gastric upset.

Side Effects and Adverse Reactions: Ulcers, occasional stomach bleeding, abdominal pain, nausea, vomiting, lack of appetite, heartburn, dizziness, headache, diarrhea, blurred vision, yellowing of skin or eyes, anemia, rash, hives, itching, respiratory distress, ringing in the ears, deafness, depression, confusion, convulsions, pain in extremities, drowsiness, lightheadedness, indigestion, constipation, bloating, flatulence, rectal bleeding, rectal pain, sleepiness, anxiety, muscle weakness, involuntary muscle movements, insomnia, confusion, fainting, heart flutters, swelling, weight gain, vaginal bleeding.

IONAMIN® (Pennwalt Pharmaceutical Division)

Generic Name: Phentermine resin

Dosage Form	Strength	Route
Capsule	15 mg	Oral
	30 mg	Oral

When Prescribed: Ionamin is a nervous system stimulant prescribed for weight reduction in individuals who cannot lose sufficient weight alone. Ionamin is usually prescribed for a short time (a few weeks) during which diet is also controlled.

Precautions and Warnings: Ionamin may have dangerous interactions with other prescription drugs. Ionamin therapy is not a substitute for diet. Prolonged use of this drug can result in dependency and withdrawal symptoms. The safe use of Ionamin during pregnancy has not been established. This drug is not recommended for use in children under 12 years of age. Ionamin may impair your ability to drive or operate dangerous machinery.

Side Effects and Adverse Reactions: Irregular heartbeat, excessive stimulation, restlessness, dizziness, insomnia, euphoria, uneasiness, shaking, headache, dryness of mouth, unpleasant taste, diarrhea, constipation, rash, impotence, change in sex drive.

ISOPTIN SR® (Knoll)

Generic Name: Verapamil Hydrochloride

Dosage Form	Strength	Route
Sustained Release Tablet	240 mg	Oral

When Prescribed: Isoptin SR is prescribed for the management of hypertension.

Precautions and Warnings: Patients with severe heart disease should not take Isoptin SR. In a small number of cases verapamil may induce low blood pressure. It is prudent to monitor liver function in patients taking verapamil and should be used with caution in those with liver or kidney problems.

Side Effects and Adverse Reactions: Constipation, dizziness, nausea, low blood pressure, headache, fatigue, rash, elevated liver enzymes.

ISORDIL® (Ives Laboratories, Inc.)

Generic Name: Isosorbide dinitrate

Dosage Form	Strength	Route
Sublingual tablet	2.5 mg	Dissolve under tongue
	5 mg	Dissolve under tongue
	10 mg	tongue
Chewable tablet	10 mg	Oral
Titradose (scored tablet)	5 mg	Oral
	10 mg	Oral
	20 mg	Oral
	30 mg	Oral
Sustained-action tablet	40 mg	Oral
Sustained-action capsule	40 mg	Oral

When Prescribed: Isordil is prescribed for the treatment of pain of coronary artery disease (angina pectoris).

Precautions and Warnings: Patients can develop a tolerance to this drug, which means that more of the drug is necessary to accomplish pain relief. The use of alcohol with this drug may cause adverse reactions.

Side Effects and Adverse Reactions: Flushing, severe persistent headache, dizziness, weakness, nausea, vomiting, restlessness, paleness, perspiration, collapse, rash, skin eruptions.

ISOSORBIDE DINITRATE

The generic name of a drug produced by numerous companies in different strengths. Also marketed as:

DILATRATE®-SR Reed and Carnrick;
ISO-BID® Geriatric;
ISORDIL® Wyeth;
ISOTRATE® Hauck;
SORBITRATE® Stuart.

Dosage Form	Strength	Route
Sublingual tablet	2.5 mg	Dissolve under tongue
	5 mg	
	10 mg	
Chewable Tablet	10 mg	Oral
Titradose (scored tabled)	5 mg	Oral
	10 mg	Oral
	20 mg	Oral
	30 mg	Oral
	40 mg	Oral
Sustained-action tablet	40 mg	Oral
Sustained-action capsule	40 mg	Oral

When Prescribed: Isosorbide dinitrate is prescribed for treatment of pain of coronary artery disease (angina pectoris).

Precautions and Warnings: Patients can develop tolerance to this drug, which means that more of the drug is necessary to accomplish pain relief. The use of alcohol with this drug may cause adverse reactions.

Side Effects and Adverse Reactions: Flushing, severe persistent headache, dizziness, weakness, nausea, vomiting, restlessness, paleness, perspiration, rash, skin eruptions.

K-DUR® (Key Pharmaceutical)

Generic Name: Potassium Chloride, USP

Dosage Form	Strength	Route
Tablet	750 mg (10 mEq)	Oral
(Extended Release)	1500 mg (20 mEq)	Oral

When Prescribed: K-Dur is prescribed to treat the deficiency of potassium in the blood.

Precautions and Warnings: Due to reports of gastric and intestinal ulceration and bleeding with time-released potassium, K-Dur should be prescribed only for those who cannot tolerate liquid or effervescent potassium. Potassium supplements taken by patients with high serum potassium risk cardiac arrest. The use of potassium salts in patients with kidney failure or problems of excretion should be closely monitored. Take each dose with meals, with a full glass of water without sucking, crushing or chewing the tablet. Safety and effectiveness of use has not been established in children.

Side Effects and Adverse Reactions: Hyperkalemia (excessive blood potassium), intestinal perforation and bleeding, ulcers, nausea, vomiting, flatulence, stomach pain, diarrhea.

KEFLEX® (Eli Lilly and Company)

Generic Name: Cephalexin monohydrate

Dosage Form	Strength	Route
Capsule	250 mg	Oral
(Pulvules®)	500 mg	Oral
Liquid	125 mg/5 ml	Oral
	250 mg/5 cc	Oral

When Prescribed: Keflex is an antibiotic prescribed for a variety of infections including those of the respiratory tract, the ear, bone, the skin, and the urogenital tract (including infection of the prostate).

Precautions and Warnings: Allergic reactions to Keflex can occur. People who are allergic to penicillin are often allergic to Keflex. Consult your physician if any side effect or adverse reaction occurs. Safety of Keflex during pregnancy has not been established.

Side Effects and Adverse Reactions: Diarrhea, nausea, vomiting, indigestion, abdominal pain, rash, hives, swelling, itching and infection of the urogenital region, dizziness, fatigue, headache, superinfection by nonsusceptible organisms.

KEFTAB® (Dista)

Generic Name: Cephalexin Hydrochloride

Dosage Form	Strength	Route
Tablet	250 mg	Oral
	500 mg	Oral

When Prescribed: Keftab is a semisynthetic antibiotic prescribed for varied infections including those of the urinary and respiratory tract, skin and bones.

Precautions and Warnings: This drug may cause allergic reactions in people who are allergic to penicillin. Keftab should be cautiously used in patients with kidney disease, pregnant women, and should be avoided by nursing mothers. Its safety and effectiveness in children has not been established.

Side Effects and Adverse Reactions: Colitis, diarrhea, rash, allergic reactions.

KENALOG® (E. R. Squibb and Sons, Inc.)

Generic Name: Triamcinolone acetonide

Dosage Form	Strength	Route
Cream	0.025% 0.1% 0.5%	Each form is applied topically
Lotion	0.025% 0.1%	to affected area
Ointment	0.025% 0.1% 0.5%	
Spray	Available in one strength only	

When Prescribed: Kenalog is a potent drug which is prescribed for topical use for relief of pain, itching, swelling and inflammation caused by various conditions such as allergic reactions.

Precautions and Warnings: Should be kept out of eyes. Kenalog should not be used extensively over large areas of the body or for extended periods of time by pregnant women.

Side Effects and Adverse Reactions: Burning, itching, irritation, dryness, hair follicle infection, excessive hair growth, acnelike eruptions, loss of skin color, dead skin, infection, loss of skin.

KLONOPIN® (Roche)

Generic Name: Clonazepam (Roche)

Dosage Form	Strength	Route
Tablet	.5 mg	Oral
	1 mg	Oral
	2 mg	Oral

When Prescribed: Klonopin is prescribed for the treatment of epileptic seizures.

Precautions and Warnings: Klonopin should not be taken by patients with a history of sensitivity to benzodiazepines, liver disease, acute narrow angle glaucoma. Klonopin can bring on grand mal seizures in patients where several types of seizures coexist. When discontinuing Klonopin gradual withdrawal is essential. Persons using this drug should not drive or operate machinery.

Side Effects and Adverse Reactions: The most frequently occurring are drowsiness, confusion, and behavior problems. Others are: abnormal eye movements, loss of voice, coma, headache, forgetfulness, hallucinations, hysteria, palpitations, swelling, rash, hair loss, chest congestion and shortness of breath, dry mouth, coated tongue, diarrhea, nausea, low blood count, liver disturbances.

KLOTRIX® (Mead Johnson Pharmaceutical Division)

Generic Name: Potassium chloride

Dosage Form	Strength	Route
Tablet	Available in one strength only	Oral

When Prescribed: Klotrix is prescribed to replace potassium in patients who, for a variety of reasons, cannot maintain normal potassium levels.

Precautions and Warnings: These tablets should be swallowed whole and never crushed or chewed to permit them to dissolve *slowly* in the system. This drug is in the form of a wax which may be observed in the stool. This is normal. Taking this medication with food may help to reduce gastrointestinal side effects.

Side Effects and Adverse Reactions: Nausea, vomiting, abdominal discomfort, diarrhea, rash, blood in vomit or stool, black vomit or stool.

K-LYTE/CL® (Mead Johnson Pharmaceutical Division)

Generic Name: Potassium chloride

Dosage Form	Strength	Route
Tablet	Available in one strength only	Oral
Powder	Available in one strength only	Oral

When Prescribed: K-Lyte/Cl is prescribed to replace potassium, an essential salt, in patients who are deficient in potassium. Potassium deficiency can result from the use of drugs that control blood pressure and for other reasons, among which is prolonged diarrhea resulting from a variety of disorders.

Precautions and Warnings: The tablet or the powder must be dissolved completely in the recommended amount of water. K-Lyte/Cl should be taken with meals and sipped slowly over a five to ten minute period.

Side Effects and Adverse Reactions: Nausea, vomiting, diarrhea, abdominal discomfort.

K-TAB® (Abbott Laboratories)

Generic Name: Potassium chloride

Dosage Form	Strength	Route
Tablet	Available in one strength only	Oral

When Prescribed: K-Tab is prescribed to replace potassium in patients who, for a variety of reasons, cannot maintain normal potassium levels.

Precautions and Warnings: The safety and efficacy of this drug in children has not been established. Gastrointestinal side effects can be reduced if this medication is taken with a meal.

Side Effects and Adverse Reactions: Vomiting, abdominal pain, abdominal distension, blood in vomit, blood in stool, black vomit, black tarry stool, diarrhea, rash.

KWELL® (Reed and Carnrick)

Generic Name: Lindane, Gamma benzene hexachloride

Dosage Form	Strength	Route
Cream	Available in one strength only	Applied directly to affected area
Shampoo	Available in one strength only	Topical, each form
Lotion	Available in one strength only	

When Prescribed: Kwell is a drug which kills parasites that live on humans. It is used for the treatment of scabies, a parasitic infection characterized by intense itching especially at night, as well as lice which live in hair on the head and in the pubic region.

Precautions and Warnings: Prolonged or repeated applications should be avoided. Avoid contact with eyes.

Side Effects and Adverse Reactions: Irritation, rash.

LANOXIN® (Burroughs Wellcome)

Generic Name: Digoxin

Dosage Form	Strength	Route
Tablet	0.125 mg	Oral
	0.25 mg	Oral
	0.5 mg	Oral
Liquid	0.05 mg/cc	Oral

When Prescribed: Lanoxin is a drug which increases the strength of the contractions of the heart. It is prescribed for patients with various forms of heart disease. It may also be used to control an irregular heartbeat.

Precautions and Warnings: Lanoxin is a potent drug which can cause serious side effects, particularly if taken in excess. Lanoxin should be taken only under the close supervision of a physician to whom any side effects or adverse reactions should be reported.

Side Effects and Adverse Reactions: Loss of appetite, excessive salivation, nausea, vomiting, diarrhea, lethargy, drowsiness, confusion, visual disturbances, irregular heartbeat, blurred vision, changes in color perceptions, headache, weakness.

LASIX® (Hoechst-Roussel Pharmaceuticals, Inc.)

Generic Name: Furosemide

Dosage Form	Strength	Route
Tablet	20 mg	Oral
	40 mg	Oral
	80 mg	Oral
Liquid	10 mg/ml	Oral

When Prescribed: Lasix is a potent drug which helps the body to pass excess water and salt, causing a prompt and copious flow of urine. It is used in treatment of heart disease, liver problems, kidney disease and high blood pressure. It is used where weaker agents are deemed not as effective.

Precautions and Warnings: Lasix is not recommended for pregnant women; however, it is safe and effective in infants and children when used as directed in the prescribing information. Lasix should be taken only under the close supervision of your physician.

Side Effects and Adverse Reactions: Abdominal pain or distension, nausea, vomiting, weakness, fatigue, dizziness, lethargy, leg cramps, loss of appetite, mental confusion, hives, itching, skin reactions, numbness, tingling of skin, blurring of vision, diarrhea, anemia, ringing in the ears, deafness, sweet taste, oral or gastric burning, swelling, headache, yellowing of skin or eyes, blood clots, thirst, increased perspiration, urinary frequency.

LEDERCILLIN VK® (Lederle)

Generic Name: Penicillin V Potassium

Dosage Form	Strength	Route
Tablet	125 mg 200,000 units	Oral
	250 mg 400,000 units	Oral
	500 mg 800,000 units	Oral
Liquid	125 mg 200,000 units	Oral
	250 mg 400,000 units	Oral

When Prescribed: Ledercillin VK is a form of penicillin which is prescribed for the treatment of mild to moderately severe infections.

Precautions and Warnings: The use of any penicillin should be discontinued and a physician consulted if any of the symptoms listed below appear.

Side Effects and Adverse Reactions: Nausea, vomiting, chest or stomach pains, diarrhea, changes in color/texture of oral mucosal membranes, skin rash, hives, chills, fever, swelling, pain in joints, fainting, superinfection by nonsusceptible organisms.

Levothyroxine Sod-(Continued)

with caution. Report the occurrences of any of the symptoms listed below immediately to your physician.

Side Effects and Adverse Reactions: Chest pains, increased pulse rate, palpitations, excessive sweating, unable to tolerate heat, nervousness or any other unusual event (signs of overactive thyroid).

LEVOTHYROXINE SOD®

This is the generic name for thyroid tablets supplied by several manufacturers, in at least 9 different strengths for easy adjustment of dosage. Also marketed as:
Synthroid® (Flint)
Levothroid® (Daniels Pharmaceutical)

Dosage Form	Strength	Route
	.025 mg	Oral
	.05 mg	Oral
	.075 mg	Oral
	.1 mg	Oral
	.125 mg	Oral
	.15 mg	Oral
	.175 mg	Oral
	.2 mg	Oral
	.3 mg	Oral

When Prescribed: Levothyroxine is prescribed for the treatment of hypothyroidism. To control symptoms you must take Levothyroxine SOD continuously. It may also be used in the treatment of goiter.

Precautions and Warnings: Levothyroxine SOD should not be used in patients with overactive thyroid, or with acute heart disease. It should not be used in patients with insufficient adrenal or by patients allergic to any of its components. The use of this drug to treat obesity is not justified. In some obese patients average doses are ineffective while larger doses may produce life-threatening toxicity. This drug should not be used for the treatment of infertility in men or women. It should be used with caution in patients with heart disease and high blood pressure. This is a potent drug and its use should be thoroughly discussed with your doctor. Thyroid-replacement medication is usually taken for life and should not be discontinued in pregnant women. But nursing mothers should use the drug

LIBRAX® (Roche Products, Inc.)

Generic Name: Chlordiazepoxide hydrochloride, clidinium bromide

Dosage Form	Strength	Route
Capsule	Available in one strength only	Oral

When Prescribed: Librax is prescribed for the relief of symptoms of an overactive gastrointestinal tract and the anxiety and tension that often accompany such disorders. It is often used, along with other drugs, in the management of ulcers.

Precautions and Warnings: Librax should not be taken with alcohol, sedatives, sleeping pills or tranquilizers. Patients using this drug should not drive or operate dangerous machinery. A physical and/or psychological dependence can occur with overuse. The use of this drug during pregnancy should almost always be avoided.

Side Effects and Adverse Reactions: Drowsiness, loss of balance, confusion, fainting, skin eruptions, swelling, menstrual irregularities, nausea, constipation, changes in sex drive, anemia, dryness of mouth, blurring of vision, difficulty in urination.

LIBRIUM® (Roche Products, Inc.)

Generic Name: Chlordiazepoxide hydrochloride

Dosage Form	Strength	Route
Capsule	5 mg	Oral
	10 mg	Oral
	25 mg	Oral
Libritab® Tablet	5 mg	Oral
	10 mg	Oral
	25 mg	Oral

When Prescribed: Librium is prescribed for a variety of emotional disorders including anxiety, tension and withdrawal symptoms of acute alcoholism. It is also prescribed to relieve the apprehension and anxiety associated with diseases.

Precautions and Warnings: Should not be combined with alcohol, sedatives, tranquilizers or sleeping pills. Persons using this drug should not drive or operate machinery. Physical and/or psychological dependence can occur with overuse. The use of Librium in pregnant women should almost always be avoided.

Side Effects and Adverse Reactions: Drowsiness, loss of balance, confusion, fainting, skin disorders, swelling, menstrual irregularities, nausea, constipation, altered sex drive, fainting, personality changes.

LIDEX® (Syntex Laboratories, Inc.)

Generic Name: Fluocinonide

Dosage Form	Strength	Route
Cream	0.05%	Topical (apply directly to affected area)
Ointment	0.05%	Topical (apply directly to affected area)

When Prescribed: Lidex is prescribed for the relief of inflammation, swelling, and itching resulting from various skin disorders.

Precautions and Warnings: Lidex is not for use in the eye. This preparation should not be used extensively by pregnant patients, in large amounts or for prolonged periods of time.

Side Effects and Adverse Reactions: Burning sensation, itching, dryness, infection of skin or hair follicles, skin eruptions, loss of pigment, skin damage.

LIMBITROL® (Roche Products, Inc.)

Generic Name: Chlordiazepoxide, amitripyline hydrochloride

Dosage Form	Strength	Route
Tablet	10–25 5–12.5	Oral

When Prescribed: Limbitrol is prescribed for the treatment of patients with moderate to severe depression associated with moderate to severe anxiety.

Precautions and Warnings: This drug should not be taken with alcohol, sleeping pills, sedatives, or tranquilizers unless directed by your physician. Patients taking Limbitrol may become drowsy. If this occurs, you should not drive or operate dangerous machinery. This drug is not recommended for pregnant women, nursing mothers, or children under 12 years of age. Prolonged use of this substance may cause psychological or physical dependance.

Side Effects and Adverse Reactions: Drowsiness, dry mouth, constipation, blurred vision, dizziness, bloating, vivid dreams, impotence, tremors, confusion, nasal congestion, loss of appetite, fatigue, weakness, restlessness, lethargy.

LITHIUM CARBONATE

The generic name for a drug produced by numerous companies in various forms and strengths. Also marketed as:
ESKALITH® Smith Kline and French;
LITHANE® Miles Pharmaceuticals;
LITHOBID® Ciba.

Dosage Form	Strength	Route
Capsule	300 mg	Oral
Tablet	300 mg	Oral

When Prescribed: Lithium carbonate is prescribed for the treatment of manic-depressive illness.

Precautions and Warnings: Lithium carbonate should not be given to pregnant or nursing women. Safety and effectiveness of this product have not been established for children under the age of 12. The salt and fluid intake should be adequate when a patient is taking this drug. Any other medication should not be taken without informing the physician, especially when the other drugs are used to treat high blood pressure.

Side Effects and Adverse Reactions: Lithium carbonate's side effects depend on its blood concentration. They can include: hand tremor, mild thirst and nausea, general discomfort, diarrhea, vomiting, drowsiness, muscle weakness, giddiness, ataxia (uncoordinated movements), blurred vision, ringing in the ears.

LOESTRIN-FE 1.5/30® (Parke Davis)

Generic Name: Norethindrone Acetate, Ethinyl, Ferrous Fumarate

Dosage Form	Strength	Route
Tablet	1 mg/20 mcg/ 75 mg	Oral

When Prescribed: Loestrin-FE 1.5/30 is an oral contraceptive prescribed for birth control.

Precautions and Warnings: Oral contraceptives are powerful and effective drugs which can have serious side effects including heart attacks, blood clots, strokes, liver tumors, gall bladder disease and high blood pressure. Safe use of this drug requires a discussion with your physician. A booklet has been prepared to provide you with additional information. Ask your doctor for this booklet. If any of the symptoms listed below are noticed, or anything unusual occurs, consult your doctor immediately. Cigarette smoking greatly increases the risk of cardiovascular side effects. Women who use this drug should not smoke.

Side Effects and Adverse Reactions: Nausea, vomiting, abdominal cramps, bloating, bleeding or spotting at times other than during menstruation, change in menstrual flow, painful and/or absence of menstruation, temporary infertility after discontinuing treatment, swelling, abnormal darkening of the skin, breast changes, including tenderness, enlargement, and secretion, weight gain or loss, change in vaginal secretion, reduction in amount of breast milk if taken after childbirth, yellowing of skin or eyes, headaches, rash, depression, vaginal infections, cramps, sensi-

LOMOTIL® (Searle and Company)

Generic Name: Diphenoxylate hydrochloride, atropine sulfate

Dosage Form	Strength	Route
Tablet	Available in one strength only	Oral
Liquid	Available in one strength only	Oral

When Prescribed: Lomotil is prescribed for the control of diarrhea. It acts by reducing intestinal movements.

Precautions and Warnings: Lomotil is not recommended for pregnant women, nursing mothers or children under the age of 2. Patients using Lomotil should not use alcohol, tranquilizers, sleeping pills or sedatives. This drug can be habit forming if overused.

Side Effects and Adverse Reactions: Dryness of mouth, dryness of skin, inability to urinate, flushing of skin, rash, abdominal discomfort, swelling of the gums, blurred vision, respiratory depression, numbness of the extremities, nausea, sedation, vomiting, headache, dizziness, drowsiness, restlessness, hives, depression, coma, lethargy, loss of appetite, euphoria, itching.

Loestrin-fe 1.5/30-(Continued)

tivity to contact lenses, visual difficulties, uncontrollable body movements, change in sex drive, change in appetite, nervousness, dizziness, increase of facial hair, loss of scalp hair, itching, skin eruptions.

LO/OVRAL® (Wyeth Laboratories)

Generic Name: Norgestrel, ethinyl estradiol

Dosage Form	Strength	Route
Tablet	Available in one strength only	Oral

When Prescribed: Lo/Ovral is an oral contraceptive which contains the same combination of estrogen and progesterone as Ovral and other birth control pills but at a reduced dosage.

Precautions and Warnings: Oral contraceptives are powerful and effective drugs which can have serious side effects including blood clots, strokes, heart attacks, liver tumors, gall bladder disease, and high blood pressure. Safe use of this drug requires a discussion with your physician. A booklet has been prepared to provide you with additional information. Ask your doctor for this booklet. If any of the symptoms listed below are noticed, or anything unusual occurs, consult your physician immediately. Cigarette smoking greatly increases the risk of cardiovascular side effects. Women who use this drug should not smoke.

Side Effects and Adverse Reactions: Nausea, vomiting, abdominal cramps, bloating, bleeding or spotting at times other than during menstruation, change in menstrual flow, pain associated with menstruation, absence of menstruation, temporary infertility after discontinuing treatment, swelling, abnormal darkening of the skin, breast changes, including tenderness, enlargement, and secretion, increase or decrease in body weight, change in vaginal secretions, reduction in amount of breast milk if

LOPRESSOR® (Geigy Pharmaceuticals)

Generic Name: Metoprolol tartrate

Dosage Form	Strength	Route
Tablets	50 mg	Oral
	100 mg	Oral

When Prescribed: Lopressor is prescribed to control high blood pressure. It acts directly on the heart to reduce heart rate and blood pressure. It may be prescribed in combination with other drugs for the reduction of blood pressure.

Precautions and Warnings: This drug should not be taken by nursing mothers.

Side Effects and Adverse Reactions: Tiredness, dizziness, depression, headache, nightmares, insomnia, shortness of breath, slow heartbeat, cold extremities, heart flutters, diarrhea, wheezing, nausea, gastric pain, constipation, gas, heartburn, itching, rash, loss of hair, visual disturbances, sore throat, hallucinations, bruising.

LOPROX® (Hoechst-Roussel Pharmaceuticals, Inc.)

Generic Name: Ciclopirox olamine

Dosage Form	Strength	Route
Cream	Available in one strength only	Topical (apply directly to affected area)

When Prescribed: Loprox is prescribed for fungal infections of the skin.

Precautions and Warnings: This preparation is not intended for use in the eyes. Inform the physician if the area of application shows signs of increased irritation, redness, itching, burning, and swelling. Avoid the use of dressings. Safety and effectiveness of this product for children below the age of 10 has not been established.

Side Effects and Adverse Reactions: Redness of skin, itching, burning, irritation.

Lo/Ovral-(Continued)

taken after childbirth, yellowing of skin or eyes, headaches, rash, depression, vaginal infections, cramps, difficulty with contact lenses, visual difficulties, uncontrollable body movements, change in sex drive, change in appetite, nervousness, dizziness, increase of facial hair, loss of scalp hair, itching, skin eruptions.

LORELCO® (Merrell Dow)

Generic Name: Probucol

Dosage Form	Strength	Route
Tablet	250 mg	Oral
	500 mg	Oral

When Prescribed: Lorelco is prescribed to lower serum cholesterol. Drug therapy should not be used routinely for the treatment of elevated cholesterol. Dietary therapy is the initial treatment of choice.

Precautions and Warnings: This is a potent drug demanding that strict attention be paid to the indications, contraindications and warnings. It should be discussed carefully and thoroughly with your physician and used only under close medical supervision. Lorelco should be used by pregnant women with great caution and avoided by nursing mothers.

Side Effects and Adverse Reactions: Acute cardiovascular disease; palpitations; chest pain; rapid heart rate; diarrhea or loose stool; gas; abdominal pain; nausea; vomiting; indigestion; gastrointestinal bleeding; headache; dizziness; numbness of extremities; tremors; insomnia; ringing, roaring, hissing noises in the ears; peripheral neuritis; rash; sweating; impotence; conjunctivitis; blurred vision; tearing of eye tissue; enlargement of goiter; fluid retention; decreased sense of taste and smell; anorexia.

LOTRIMIN® (Schering Corporation)

Generic Name: Clotrimazole

Dosage Form	Strength	Route
Cream	1%	Topical (apply directly to the affected area)
Solution	1%	Topical (apply directly to the affected area)

When Prescribed: Lotrimin is an antifungal agent prescribed to treat skin infections caused by various fungal agents.

Precautions and Warnings: This preparation is not intended for use in the eye.

Side Effects and Adverse Reactions: Reddening of the skin, stinging, blistering, peeling, swelling, itching, rash, irritation.

LOTRISONE® (Schering Corporation)

Generic Name: Clotrimazole, beta-methasone dipropionate

Dosage Form	Strength	Route
Cream	Available in one strength only	Topical (apply directly to affected area)

When Prescribed: Lotrisone is prescribed to treat fungal infections of the skin associated with inflammation.

Precautions and Warnings: It should be used with caution when used for a prolonged period of time on large surface areas or with occlusive dressings. Patients should inform the physician of any type of abnormal skin reaction. Contact of this medication with the eyes should be avoided. The drug's safety and efficacy have not been established for pregnant women and nursing mothers. It should be stored at temperatures between 2° and 30° C, or 35.6° and 86° F.

Side Effects and Adverse Reactions: Skin rashes, peeling of skin, edema, irritation, burning, itching, dryness, decrease in pigmentation, secondary infections.

LOZOL® (USV Laboratories)

Generic Name: Indapamide

Dosage Form	Strength	Route
Tablet	2.5 mg	Oral

When Prescribed: Lozol is prescribed for treatment of high blood pressure.

Precautions and Warnings: Lozol may decrease the body's potassium level, an adequate amount of which is necessary for muscle movement. The use of other drugs along with Lozol should have your physician's consent.

Side Effects and Adverse Reactions: Headache, dizziness, fatigue, loss of energy, muscle cramps, nervousness, anxiety, tension, insomnia, drowsiness, constipation, blurred vision, gastric irritation, anorexia, rash, hives, increase in blood sugar level.

LUDIOMIL® (Ciba Pharmaceutical Company)

Generic Name: Maprotiline hydrochloride

Dosage Form	Strength	Route
Tablets	25 mg	Oral
	50 mg	

When Prescribed: Ludiomil is prescribed for the treatment of depression and anxiety associated with depression.

Precautions and Warnings: Ludiomil should not be taken with alcohol, sleeping pills, tranquilizers, or other depressants without the consent of your physician. If drowsiness occurs, you should not drive or operate dangerous machinery. The safe use of this drug in people under 18 years of age has not been established.

Side Effects and Adverse Reactions: Changes in blood pressure, rapid heartbeat, heart flutters, fainting, nervousness, anxiety, insomnia, agitation, confusion, hallucinations, disorientation, delusions, restlessness, nightmares, hyperactivity, decrease in memory, feelings of unreality, drowsiness, dizziness, tremor, abnormal sensation, ringing in the ears, dry mouth, constipation, blurred vision, urinary problems, rash, itching, increased sensitivity to sunlight, swelling, fever, nausea, vomiting, heartburn, diarrhea, bitter taste, abdominal cramps, difficulty in swallowing, change in sex drive, impotence, weakness, fatigue, headache, yellowing of skin or eyes, changes in weight, excessive sweating, flushing of skin, urinary frequency, increased salivation, nasal congestion.

LURIDE® (Colgate-Hoyt Laboratories)

Generic Name: Sodium fluoride

Dosage Form	Strength	Route
Liquid	4 mg fluoride/ml	Oral
Chewable	.25 mg	Oral
Tablet	.5 mg	Oral
	1 mg	Oral

When Prescribed: It has been established that ingestion of water which contains fluoride during the period of tooth development results in a significant decrease in the incidence of dental cavities. It is prescribed for children from birth to 3 years and older living in an area where drinking water fluoride levels are less than 0.7 parts per million.

Precautions and Warnings: Do not use Luride in an area where the drinking water contains more than 0.7 parts fluoride per million. Do not use with milk or other dairy products.

Side Effects and Adverse Reactions: Allergic rash has been reported rarely.

MACRODANTIN® (Norwich-Eaton Pharmaceuticals)

Generic Name: Nitrofurantoin macrocrystals

Dosage Form	Strength	Route
Capsule	25 mg	Oral
	50 mg	Oral
	100 mg	Oral

When Prescribed: Macrodantin is an antibacterial agent for specific urinary tract infections of the kidney and bladder.

Precautions and Warnings: Macrodantin usually is not prescribed for pregnant women at term or for lactating mothers.

Side Effects and Adverse Reactions: Loss of appetite, nausea, vomiting, diarrhea, cutaneous eruptions, rash, itching, swelling, anemia, chills, fever, yellowing of the skin or eyes, fainting, chest congestion, headache, dizziness, abnormal eye movements, loss of balance, drowsiness, depression, muscle aches, loss of hair, superinfection by nonsusceptible organisms.

MATERNA 1-60® (Lederle Laboratories)

Generic Name: Phosphorus-free vitamins and minerals

Dosage Form	Strength	Route
Tablet	Available in one strength only	Oral

When Prescribed: Materna 1-60 is a vitamin and mineral supplement prescribed for use during pregnancy and lactation.

Precautions and Warnings: Do not exceed recommended dosage.

Side Effects and Adverse Reactions: This drug is well tolerated. No side effects are listed.

MAXITROL® (Alcon Inc.)

Generic Name: Neomycin sulfate, dexamethasone, polymixin B sulfate

Dosage Form	Strength	Route
Ophthalmic Suspension (eye drops)	Available in one strength only	Eye Drops

When Prescribed: Maxitrol is a combination of antiinfective and steroid. It is prescribed for infection and inflammation responsive to the steroid.

Precautions and Warnings: Maxitrol cannot be used as an injection. Prolonged use of this product may result in glaucoma with damage to nerve of the eye, defects in the vision field, and an increase in the chances of secondary infections.

Side Effects and Adverse Reactions: Allergy, sensitization, cataract formation, possibility of glaucoma, delayed wound healing, secondary infection.

MECLIZINE The generic name for a drug produced by numerous companies in different strengths. Also marketed as: BONINE® (Pfipharmecs); RU-VERT-M® (Reid-Rowell, Inc.); ANTIVERT® (Roerig).

Dosage Form	Strength	Route
Tablet	12.5 mg	Oral
	25 mg	Oral
	50 mg	Oral
Tablet (chewable)	25 mg	Oral

When Prescribed: Meclizine is an antihistamine which has been shown to be effective in the management of nausea, vomiting, and dizziness associated with motion sickness. It is possibly effective, though not proven, in management of dizziness associated with diseases of the vestibular (balance) system.)

Precautions and Warnings: Meclizine is not recommended during pregnancy or for women who may become pregnant while taking the drug, nor is it recommended for preadolescent children. Because drowsiness may occur on occasions, patients should not drive cars or operate dangerous machinery.

Side Effects and Adverse Reactions: Drowsiness, dry mouth and, on rare occasions, blurred vision.

MECLOMEN® (Parke-Davis and Company)

Generic Name: Meclofenamate sodium

Dosage Form	Strength	Route
Capsule	50 mg 100 mg	Oral

When Prescribed: Meclomen is prescribed for the relief of symptoms in rheumatoid arthritis and in osteoarthritis.

Precautions and Warnings: Meclomen can be taken with meals or with an antacid to help avoid stomach upset. This drug is not recommended for pregnant women, nursing mothers, or children under the age of 14.

Side Effects and Adverse Reactions: Diarrhea, nausea, vomiting, gastrointestinal disorders, abdominal pain, heartburn, gas, loss of appetite, constipation, stomach pain, ulcers, swelling, rash, hives, itching, headache, dizziness, ringing in the ears, black tarry stools, blood in vomit, dark vomit, heart flutters, depression, fatigue, abnormal sensations, insomnia, blurred vision, taste disturbances, urinary problems.

MEDROL® (The Upjohn Company)

Generic Name: Methylprednisolone

Dosage Form	Strength	Route
Tablet	2 mg	Oral
	4 mg	Oral
	8 mg	Oral
	16 mg	Oral
	24 mg	Oral
	32 mg	Oral
Dosepak™	4 mg	Oral

When Prescribed: Medrol is the manmade equivalent of a substance produced naturally in the body by the adrenal glands. The main action of Medrol is to reduce inflammation and swelling. Medrol is prescribed for a variety of reasons including glandular disorders, rheumatic and arthritic disorders, diseases of connective tissues, skin diseases, allergies, eye disorders, respiratory diseases, blood disorders, swelling, meningitis, tuberculosis, gastrointestinal diseases, swelling from dental work.

Precautions and Warnings: Mothers taking Medrol should not nurse. Patients on Medrol therapy should not receive smallpox or other vaccinations. Prolonged use of Medrol may cause psychological and/or physical dependence and subsequent withdrawal symptoms.

Side Effects and Adverse Reactions: Fluid retention, swelling, muscle weakness, ulcer, stomach irritation, slow wound healing, increased sweating, allergic skin reactions, convulsions, dizziness, headache, menstrual irregularities, suppression of growth in children, bulging of the eyes.

MELLARIL® (Sandoz Pharmaceuticals)

Generic Name: Thioridazine hydrochloride

Dosage Form	Strength	Route
Tablet	10 mg	Oral
	15 mg	Oral
	25 mg	Oral
	50 mg	Oral
	100 mg	Oral
	150 mg	Oral
	200 mg	Oral
Liquid	30 mg/ml	Oral
	100 mg/ml	Oral

When Prescribed: Mellaril is prescribed for management of certain emotional disorders which are characterized by abnormal agitation, aggressiveness, or excitement. It is often prescribed for overaggressive children. It can also be prescribed for use in alcohol withdrawal, severe pain and senility.

Precautions and Warnings: This drug may impair mental and/or physical abilities required for performance of hazardous tasks such as operating machinery or driving motor vehicles. Mellaril should not be taken with alcohol, tranquilizers, sleeping pills or sedatives.

Side Effects and Adverse Reactions: Drowsiness, uncoordinated movements, tremors, confusion, hyperactivity, lethargy, psychotic reactions, restlessness, headache, dryness of mouth, blurred vision, constipation, nausea, vomiting, diarrhea, nasal stuffiness, paleness, breast enlargement, lack of menstruation, inhibition of ejaculation, false positive pregnancy tests, swelling, skin eruptions, hives, loss of appetite, anemia, fever, yellowing of skin or eyes, heart failure, abnormal movements of the face, tongue or jaw, loss of visual acuity, brownish coloring of vision, impairment of night vision, urinary difficulties.

MEPROBAMATE
The generic name for a drug produced by numerous companies in various forms and strengths. Also marketed as:
EQUANIL®, Wyeth;
KESSO-BAMATE®, McKesson;
MEPROSPAN®, Wallace;
MEPROTABS®, Wallace;
MILTOWN®, Wallace;
SK-BAMATE®, Smith Kline and French.

Generic Name: Meprobamate

Dosage Form	Strength	Route
Tablet	200 mg	Oral
	400 mg	Oral

When Prescribed: Meprobamate is prescribed for the relief of anxiety and tension, often in patients with various disease states which lead to anxiety and tension. It is also used to promote sleep in tense, anxious patients.

Precautions and Warnings: Overuse of this drug can lead to physical and/or psychological dependence. Sudden withdrawal after prolonged and excessive use may cause adverse reactions. Meprobamate may impair the mental or physical abilities required for the performance of potentially hazardous tasks such as driving or operating machinery. Should not be taken with alcohol, tranquilizers, sedatives, or sleeping pills. The safe use of this drug in pregnancy has not been established.

Side Effects and Adverse Reactions: Drowsiness, loss of balance, dizziness, slurred speech, headache, weakness, tingling, crawling skin, inability of eyes to adapt to changing light, euphoria, stimulation, excitement, nausea, vomiting, diarrhea, flutters of the heart, increased heart rate, fainting, itching, rash, hives, anemia, swelling, fever, chills, frequent urination, inability to urinate, darkening of urine.

METRONIDAZOLE The generic name for a drug produced by numerous companies in two different strengths. Also marketed as: PROTOSTAT® Ortho; SK-METRONIDAZOLE® Smith Kline & French; SATRIC® Savage; FLAGYL® Searle; METRYL® Lemmon.

Generic Name: Metronidazole hydrochloride

Dosage Form	Strength	Route
Tablet	250 mg	Oral
	500 mg	Oral

When Prescribed: Metronidazole is prescribed for the treatment of certain infections (trichomoniasis) of the genital tract in both males and females. It is also prescribed for the treatment of dysentery (amoebic dysentery) and liver abscess caused by amoebas.

Precautions and Warnings: Alcoholic beverages should not be consumed during metronidazole therapy because abdominal cramps, vomiting, and flushing may occur. This drug is not recommended for pregnant women or nursing mothers. If you have any central nervous system disorders, inform your physician about this before starting the therapy.

Side Effects and Adverse Reactions: Nausea, headache, loss of appetite, vomiting, diarrhea, heartburn, cramps, constipation, unpleasant metallic taste, furry tongue, sore throat, dizziness, incoordination, loss of balance, numbness, crawling skin, joint pain, confusion, irritability, depression, insomnia, rash, weakness, hives, dryness of mouth, itching, painful urination, painful sexual intercourse, decreased sex drive, frequent urination, nasal congestion, pus in urine, inflammation of bowel, darkening of urine, superinfection by nonsusceptible organisms.

MEVACOR® (Merick Sharp and Dohme)

Generic Name: Lovastatin (MSD)

Dosage Form	Strength	Route
Tablets	20 mg	Oral
	40 mg	Oral

When Prescribed: Mevacor is prescribed for lowering elevated serum cholesterol when dietary restrictions alone have proven inadequate.

Precautions and Warnings: Before using Mevacor an attempt to reduce cholesterol levels through diet, exercise, and weight reduction should be made. Mevacor should not be taken by patients with liver disease, nor pregnant and lactating mothers. Liver function tests should be performed prior to treatment, every 4–6 weeks during the first 15 months and periodically thereafter in all patients. This drug should be used cautiously by patients who drink alcohol heavily or have a history of liver disease. Patients receiving lovastatin and erythromycin should be carefully monitored by the physician. The combined use of lovastatin with a group of lipid-lowering drugs known as fibrates should be avoided. When lovastatin is combined with other lipid-lowering drugs, the physician should carefully monitor patients for muscle pain, tenderness, or weakness. Mevacor should be avoided by patients with acute infection, major surgery, trauma, and uncontrolled seizures. Report immediately to your doctor any unexplained muscular pain or weakness.

Side Effects and Adverse Reactions: Liver disease, muscular pain and weakness, fever, malaise, hepatitis, anorexia,

112

MICRO-K® (A. H. Robins Company)

Generic Name: Potassium chloride

Dosage Form	Strength	Route
Capsule	600 mg	Oral
	750 mg	Oral

When Prescribed: Micro-K is prescribed to replace potassium, an essential salt, for patients who are deficient in potassium. Potassium deficiency can result from the use of drugs that control blood pressure, among other reasons.

Precautions and Warnings: Because of reports of intestinal and gastric ulceration and bleeding, with Micro-K and other slow-release potassium chloride preparations, these drugs should be reserved for those patients who cannot tolerate or refuse to take liquid or effervescent potassium preparations and for patients who have a problem following the instructions given for taking these preparations.

Side Effects and Adverse Reactions: Nausea, vomiting, diarrhea, abdominal discomfort, intestinal bleeding.

Mevacor-(Continued)

vomiting, pancreatitis, swelling of the mouth, loss of hair, fluid retention, depression, insomnia.

MICRONASE® (The Upjohn Company)

Generic Name: Glyburide

Dosage Form	Strength	Route
Tablet	1.25 mg	Oral
	2.5 mg	Oral
	5 mg	Oral

When Prescribed: Micronase is prescribed for diabetes (diabetes mellitus) to control the blood sugar levels in addition to diet. It is prescribed after a sufficient trial of dietary therapy has proved unsatisfactory. Micronase can replace the need for insulin by helping to release the body's own insulin.

Precautions and Warnings: Blood and urine glucose should be monitored periodically while using Micronase. The effect of decreasing blood-sugar levels can be potentiated by other drugs. Inform your physician before starting any other medication. Drinking alcohol can result in severe vomiting and abdominal cramps. Micronase should be used during pregnancy only if the potential benefit justifies the potential risk to the fetus and should be discontinued at least one month prior to the expected delivery date. Safety and effectiveness for children's use of this drug has not been established. Micronase does not replace the need to restrict diet.

Side Effects and Adverse Reactions: Jaundice, nausea, heartburn, skin rashes, different types of anemia, hypoglycemia (low blood sugar levels), diarrhea, constipation, abdominal pain, gas, itching, weakness, fatigue, loss of balance, drowsiness, dizziness, depression, headache.

MIDRIN® (Carnrick Laboratories)

Generic Name: Isometheptene mucate, dichloral phenazone, acetaminophen

Dosage Form	Strength	Route
Capsule	Available in one strength only	Oral

When Prescribed: Midrin is prescribed for relief of tension and vascular headache and is possibly effective in the treatment of migraine headache.

Precautions and Warnings: Midrin should not be used by patients suffering from renal disease, high blood pressure, or heart disease, or those using certain antidepressants.

Side Effects and Adverse Reactions: Dizziness, skin rash.

MINIPRESS® (Pfizer Laboratories Division)

Generic Name: Prazosin hydrochloride

Dosage Form	Strength	Route
Capsule	1 mg	Oral
	2 mg	Oral
	5 mg	Oral

When Prescribed: Minipress is prescribed to reduce blood pressure in patients with high blood pressure. It may be prescribed as the sole agent or in combination with other agents for the management of high blood pressure.

Precautions and Warnings: Lowering of blood pressure (the intended effect of the drug) can lead to fainting associated with changes in posture. For example, after getting up from a chair, you may experience lightheadedness or fainting. This is more likely to occur when Minipress therapy is just starting.

Side Effects and Adverse Reactions: Dizziness, headache, drowsiness, lack of energy, weakness, heart flutters, fainting, nausea, vomiting, diarrhea, constipation, abdominal upset, swelling, breathing difficulties, rapid heartbeat, nervousness, loss of balance, depression, abnormal skin sensation, rash, itching, urinary difficulties, impotence, blurred vision, red eyes, ringing in ears, dry mouth, nasal congestion.

MINOCIN® (Lederle Laboratories)

Generic Name: Minocycline hydrochloride

Dosage Form	Strength	Route
Capsule	50 mg	Oral
	100 mg	Oral
Syrup	50 mg/5 ml	Oral

When Prescribed: Minocin is a derivative of tetracycline, an effective antibiotic prescribed for many different types of infection. It is often used in place of penicillin in patients who are allergic to penicillin.

Precautions and Warnings: Minocin should not be taken by people overly sensitive to tetracycline. If any of the side effects listed below occur, consult your physician immediately. This drug can interfere with tooth development and therefore is not recommended for pregnant women, infants, or children under the age of 8. Antacids will impair absorption.

Side Effects and Adverse Reactions: Exaggerated sunburn, superinfection by nonsusceptible organisms, loss of appetite, nausea, vomiting, diarrhea, difficulty in swallowing, stomach pains, skin rash, hives, swelling, dizziness, fainting.

MODURETIC® (Merck Sharp and Dohme)

Generic Name: Amiloride hydrochloride, hydrochlorothiazide

Dosage Form	Strength	Route
Tablet	Available in one strength only	Oral

When Prescribed: Moduretic is prescribed for the treatment of high blood pressure or for congestive heart failure.

Precautions and Warnings: The safety and efficacy of this drug in children has not been established. Mothers should not nurse while taking Moduretic. This drug should be taken with food.

Side Effects and Adverse Reactions: Headache, weakness, fatigue, tiredness, depression, chest pain, back pain, heart flutters, rapid heartbeat, arm pain, nausea, loss of appetite, diarrhea, gastrointestinal pain, abdominal pain, constipation, blood in stool or vomit, black stool or vomit, gas, rash, itching, flushing of skin, leg aches, muscle cramps, joint pain, dizziness, altered sensation in skin, numbness, loss of balance, insomnia, nervousness, sleepiness, mental confusion, breathing difficulties, bad taste, visual disturbances, nasal congestion, impotence, urinary problems.

MONISTAT® 7 (Ortho Pharmaceuticals)

Generic Name: Miconazole nitrate

Dosage Form	Strength	Route
Cream	Available in one strength only	Intra-vaginal
Vaginal Suppository		Intra-vaginal

When Prescribed: Monistat is prescribed for "yeast" (or fungal) infections of the skin and of the mucous membranes of the vagina.

Precautions and Warnings: If irritation or sensitivity occurs, discontinue use and consult your physician.

Side Effects and Adverse Reactions: Burning, itching, irritation, pelvic cramps, hives, skin rash, headache.

MONISTAT DUAL-PACK® (Ortho Pharmaceutical Corporation)

Generic Name: Miconazole nitrate

Dosage Form	Strength	Route
Cream and Vaginal Suppository	Available in one strength only	Intra-vaginal

When Prescribed: Monistat Dual-Pack is a comparatively new combination of suppository and cream together. Previously both of these dosage forms were available separately. It is prescribed for the local treatment of candidiasis (a fungal infection).

Precautions and Warnings: Effectiveness of Monistat vaginal suppository and cream has not been established in diabetics. Monistat cream is for external use only. Avoid introduction of cream to the eyes. Monistat should not be used in the first trimester of pregnancy.

Side Effects and Adverse Reactions: Vaginal burning, itching, irritation, softening of tissue at the site of application, skin rash, cramps, headache, allergic reactions.

MONISTAT-DERM® (Ortho Pharmaceutical Corporation)

Generic Name: Miconazole nitrate

Dosage Form	Strength	Route
Cream	2%	Topical (apply directly to affected area)
Lotion	2%	

When Prescribed: Monistat-Derm is prescribed for the treatment of tinea pedis (athlete's foot) and other infections due to tinea and yeastlike fungus.

Precautions and Warnings: Monistat-Derm should be discontinued if a reaction occurs such as itching or irritation. Monistat-Derm should not be introduced in the eyes.

Side Effects and Adverse Reactions: Irritation, burning, allergic reaction, maceration.

MONISTAT-3® (Ortho Pharmaceutical Corporation)

Generic Name: Miconazole nitrate

Dosage Form	Strength	Route
Vaginal Suppository	Available in one strength only	Intra-vaginal

When Prescribed: Monistat-3 contains only 3 suppositories. It is prescribed for the local treatment of candidiasis (a fungal infection).

Precautions and Warnings: Effectiveness of Monistat-3 has not been established in diabetic patients. Should not be used in the first trimester of pregnancy.

Side Effects and Adverse Reactions: Vaginal burning, itching or irritation, cramps, headache, hives, skin rashes.

MOTRIN® (The Upjohn Company)

Generic Name: Ibuprofen

Dosage Form	Strength	Route
Tablet	300 mg	Oral
	400 mg	Oral
	600 mg	Oral
	800 mg	Oral

When Prescribed: Motrin is prescribed to relieve the pain and inflammation of arthritis. Motrin is as effective as aspirin for the long-term management of pain and inflammation but usually is better tolerated in terms of stomach upset and irritation.

Precautions and Warnings: Ingestion of Motrin is not recommended during pregnancy, or for nursing mothers. The use of aspirin with Motrin may reduce the effectiveness of the drug.

Side Effects and Adverse Reactions: Nausea, chest pains, heartburn, diarrhea, constipation or gastric pain, abdominal cramps or pain, vomiting, indigestion, constipation, bloating, gas, dizziness, headache, nervousness, rash, ringing in the ears, decreased appetite, depression, insomnia, visual disturbances, nightmares, fever, itching.

MYCELEX-G® (Miles Pharmaceuticals)

Generic Name: Clotrimazole

Dosage Form	Strength	Route
Cream	1%	Intra-vaginal
Suppository	100 mg	Intra-vaginal
Suppository	500 mg	Intra-vaginal

When Prescribed: Mycelex-G is prescribed for local treatment of vaginal candidiasis (fungal infection).

Precaution and Warnings: Because of the lack of information, it is suggested that Mycelex-G not be used in the first trimester of pregnancy. Use of this product in the second and third trimesters is considered safe.

Side Effects and Adverse Reactions: Vaginal burning, itching, lower abdominal cramps, slight urinary frequency, burning or irritation in the sexual partner.

MYCOLOG® (E. R. Squibb & Sons)

Generic Name: Nystatin, neomycin sulfate, gramicidin, triamcinolone acetonide

Dosage Form	Strength	Route
Cream and Ointment	Available in one strength only	Applied directly to problem area

When Prescribed: Mycolog is a topical cream that provides rapid, complete, often prolonged control of symptoms of inflammation of the skin, infections of the skin and itching of the skin. Mycolog is a combination of an antifungal agent, antibacterial agents, and a corticosteroid.

Precautions and Warnings: Mycolog should not be used extensively or for prolonged periods in pregnant patients. This preparation is not intended for use in the eyes.

Side Effects and Adverse Reactions: Burning, itching, irritation, dryness, hair follicle infections, excessive hair growth, skin eruptions, loss of pigmentation, peeling or flaking skin, superinfection by nonsusceptible organisms.

MYCOLOG II® (E. R. Squibb & Sons)

Generic Name: Nystatin, triamcinolone acetonide

Dosage Form	Strength	Route
Cream and Ointment	Available in one strength only	Topical (apply directly to affected area)

When Prescribed: Mycolog II is prescribed for the treatment of skin candidiasis.

Precautions and Warnings: Avoid contact with the eyes. Patients should not use this medication for any disorder other than that for which it was prescribed. The treated skin area should not be bandaged or otherwise covered or wrapped. Patients should report any signs of local adverse reactions. Parents of pediatric patients should be advised not to use tight-fitting diapers or plastic pants on a child being treated in the diaper area. Mycolog II should not be used extensively on pregnant patients in large amounts or for prolonged periods of time.

Side Effects and Adverse Reactions: Burning, itching, irritation, dryness, acne eruptions, maceration of skin, secondary infections.

MYCOSTATIN® (E. R. Squibb & Sons)

Generic Name: Nystatin

Dosage Form	Strength	Route
Vaginal tablet	Each form is available in one strength only	Intravaginal
Cream		Topical
Ointment		Topical
Tablet		Oral
Liquid		Oral

When Prescribed: Mycostatin is prescribed for the control of fungus (yeast) infections.

Precautions and Warnings: Mycostatin should not be used by patients with a sensitivity to the drug.

Side Effects and Adverse Reactions: Large doses of the oral forms of Mycostatin may produce diarrhea, gastrointestinal distress, nausea, vomiting.

NALDECON® (Bristol Laboratories)

Generic Name: Phenylpropanolamine hydrochloride, phenylephrine hydrochloride, phenyltoloxamine citrate, chlorpheniramine maleate

Dosage Form	Strength	Route
Tablet	Available in one strength only	Oral
Liquid	Available in one strength only	Oral
Pediatric drops	Available in one strength only	Oral
Pediatric syrup	Available in one strength only	Oral

When Prescribed: Naldecon is prescribed for the relief of symptoms of colds and other upper respiratory infections, sinus infections, hay fever and allergies.

Precautions and Warnings: This drug may cause drowsiness. Do not drive or operate machinery while taking this drug.

Side Effects and Adverse Reactions: Rash, hives, anemia, drowsiness, lassitude, giddiness, dryness of mouth or nose, painful urination, elevated blood pressure, irregular heartbeat, headache, faintness, dizziness, ringing in the ears, loss of appetite, nausea, vomiting, diarrhea, constipation.

NALFON® (Dista Products Company)

Generic Name: Fenoprofen calcium

Dosage Form	Strength	Route
Capsule	300 mg	Oral
Tablet	200 mg	Oral
	600 mg	Oral

When Prescribed: Nalfon is prescribed for the relief of pain and inflammation from arthritis. It is as effective as aspirin in reducing pain and inflammation but is usually better tolerated in the stomach.

Precautions and Warnings: This drug is not recommended for pregnant women or for nursing mothers. Nalfon should be taken thirty minutes before or two hours after a meal.

Side Effects and Adverse Reactions: Indigestion, constipation, nausea, abdominal pain, loss of appetite, blood in stool, diarrhea, gas, dry mouth, itching, rash, increased sweating, hives, sleepiness, dizziness, tremors, confusion, insomnia, ringing in the ears, blurred vision, decreased ability to hear, heart flutters, rapid heartbeat, headache, nervousness, weakness, breathing difficulties, swelling, fatigue, mood depression, urinary difficulties.

NAPHCON-A® (Alcon Inc.)

Generic Name: Naphazoline hydrochloride, pheniramine maleate

Dosage Form	Strength	Route
Ophthalmic Solution (eye drop)	Available in one strength only	Eye Drop

When Prescribed: Naphcon-A is prescribed for the relief of ocular (eye) irritation and/or congestion or for the treatment of allergic or inflammatory eye conditions.

Precautions and Warnings: Naphcon-A should be used with caution by elderly patients who suffer from heart disease or are diabetic. To prevent contamination, the dropper should not touch the eyelid or surrounding areas.

Side Effects and Adverse Reactions: Increase in internal eye pressure, dilation of pupil, visual disturbance, increase in blood pressure, increase in blood sugar level.

NAPROSYN® (Syntex)

Generic Name: Naproxen

Dosage Form	Strength	Route
Tablet	250 mg	Oral
	375 mg	Oral
	500 mg	Oral
Suspension	125 mg	Oral

When Prescribed: Naprosyn is prescribed for the treatment of rheumatoid arthritis, osteoarthritis, juvenile arthritis, ankylosing spondylitis, tendinitis and bursitis, acute gout, painful menstruation, and for the relief of mild pain.

Precautions and Warnings: Gastrointestinal bleeding, ulceration, and perforation can occur without warning. Naprosyn should not be used with Anaprox. Naprosyn can induce kidney failure and should be used with caution in patients with poor kidney function, cirrhosis, and the elderly. The safe use of this drug during pregnancy has not been established. It should be avoided by nursing mothers.

Side Effects and Adverse Reactions: Jaundice, hepatitis, drowsiness, headache, lightheadedness, dizziness, vertigo, insomnia, constipation, heartburn, abdominal pain, nausea, inflammation of the mouth, itching, skin eruptions and bruising, sweating, hearing and visual disturbances, palpitations, congestive heart failure, shortness of breath, thirst, kidney disease, vomiting, bloody stool, low white blood cell count, rash, sensitivity to sunlight, menstrual disturbances, chills and fever, anemia, cognitive disturbances, inflamed blood vessels.

NASALCROM® (Fisons Corporation)

Generic Name: Cromolyn sodium

Dosage Form	Strength	Route
Nasal Solution	Available in one strength only	Nasal Inhalation

When Prescribed: Nasalcrom is prescribed for the prevention and treatment of the symptoms of allergic inflammation of nasal mucosa.

Precautions and Warnings: Some patients may experience transient nasal stinging and/or sneezing immediately following inhalation of Nasalcrom. Except in rare occurrences, these experiences have not caused discontinuation of therapy. This drug should be used during pregnancy only if clearly needed. Caution should be exercised when Nasalcrom is administered to nursing women. Safety and effectiveness for children below the age of 6 have not been established.

Side Effects and Adverse Reactions: Nasal stinging, sneezing, nasal burning, nasal irritation, headaches, bad taste.

NASALIDE® (Syntex Laboratories, Inc.)

Generic Name: Flunisolide

Dosage Form	Strength	Route
Nasal Solution Spray	Available in one strength only	Inhalation

When Prescribed: Nasalide is prescribed for relief of symptoms of seasonal inflammation of nasal mucous membranes when effectiveness of or tolerance to conventional treatment is unsatisfactory.

Precautions and Warnings: Nasalide should not be used in the presence of untreated localized infection involving nasal mucosa. It should not be continued beyond three weeks in the absence of significant symptomatic improvement.

Side Effects and Adverse Reactions: Nasal mucosal burning and stinging, nasal congestion, sneezing, nasal irritation, watery eyes, sore throat, nausea, vomiting, headaches, loss of sense of smell and taste.

NAVANE® (Roerig)

Generic Name: Thiothixene

Dosage Form	Strength	Route
Capsule	1 mg 2 mg 5 mg 10 mg 20 mg	Oral
Liquid	Liquid comes in one strength. Dose is determined by a calibrated dropper.	Oral

When Prescribed: Navane is prescribed for the management of certain mental disorders.

Precautions and Warnings: The safe use of this drug in pregnancy has not been established. Navane should not be taken by nursing mothers or children under 12 years of age. This drug should not be taken with alcohol, sleeping pills, sedatives or tranquilizers unless specifically directed by your physician. If drowsiness occurs, you should not drive or operate dangerous machinery.

Side Effects and Adverse Reactions: Rapid heartbeat, lightheadedness, fainting, drowsiness, restlessness, agitation, insomnia, seizures, abnormal body movements, abnormal facial movements or expressions, rash, itching, hives, increased sensitivity to sunlight, breast enlargement, lactation, menstrual difficulties, dry mouth, blurred vision, nasal congestion, constipation, increased sweating, increased salivation, impotence, visual difficulties, fever, loss of appetite, nausea, vomiting, diarrhea, increase in appetite, weight gain, weakness, fatigue, excessive thirst, swelling.

NEODECADRON® OPHTHALMIC
SOLUTION (Merck Sharp and Dohme)

Generic Name: Dexamethasone sodium phosphate, neomycin

Dosage Form	Strength	Route
Liquid	Available in one strength only	Eye Drops

When Prescribed: Neodecadron ophthalmic solution is a potent drug which is prescribed for treatment of inflammation of the eye and surrounding tissue. It is effective in reducing inflammation often associated with infection. This preparation contains a steroid to reduce inflammation and an antibiotic, as well.

Precautions and Warnings: If used for prolonged periods, eye examinations should be performed frequently. This preparation should not be used for prolonged periods by pregnant patients.

Side Effects and Adverse Reactions: Increased eye pressure, nerve damage, visual defects, cataracts, secondary infection, stinging, burning.

NEOSPORIN® OPHTHALMIC
SOLUTION (Burroughs Wellcome Company)

Generic Name: Polymyxin B-neomycin gramicidin

Dosage Form	Strength	Route
Liquid	Available in one strength only	Eye Drops

When Prescribed: Neosporin is prescribed for the short-term treatment of superficial infections of the eye.

Precautions and Warnings: The solution as contained in the bottle is sterile. Patients should use caution in placing the drops into the eye so as not to contaminate the dropper. This is best done by preventing the tip from touching the eyelid or surrounding areas.

Side Effects and Adverse Reactions: Sensitization of the skin or surface of the eye.

NICORETTE® (Lakeside Pharmaceuticals)

Generic Name: Nicotine polacrilex

Dosage Form	Strength	Route
Gum	2 mg	Oral

When Prescribed: Nicorette is prescribed as a temporary aid to the cigarette smoker seeking to give up his or her smoking habit while participating in a behavior modification program under medical supervision.

Precautions and Warnings: Patients with heart disease such as arrhythmia or angina pectoris, pregnant women, and nursing mothers should not use Nicorette. It should also not be used by non-smokers.

Side Effects and Adverse Reactions: Injury to oral mucosa or teeth, jaw aches, excess salivation, gastric distress, nausea, vomiting, mouth and throat soreness, hiccups.

NITRO-BID® (Marion Laboratories, Inc.)

Generic Name: Nitroglycerin

Dosage Form	Strength	Route
Capsule	2.5 mg	Oral
(plateau	6.5 mg	Oral
capsule®)	9.0 mg	Oral
prolonged action		

When Prescribed: Nitro-Bid is prescribed for the relief of angina pectoris (chest pain) which often accompanies heart conditions such as coronary artery disease. It acts by increasing the blood flow to the heart muscle.

Precautions and Warnings: While some nitroglycerin preparations are meant to be dissolved under the tongue, Nitro-bid capsules should be swallowed. Nitro-bid is not intended for immediate relief of angina attacks but meant to produce relief for 8 to 12 hours.

Side Effects and Adverse Reactions: Severe and persistent headaches, cutaneous flushing, dizziness, weakness, nausea, vomiting, rash. Adverse reactions are made worse if alcohol is consumed.

NITRO-DUR® II (Key Pharmaceuticals Inc.)

Generic Name: Nitroglycerin

Dosage Form	Strength	Route
Skin Patch	2.5 mg/24 hrs (5 cm²)	Local Apply to the skin
	5 mg/24 hrs (10 cm²)	
	7.5 mg/24 hrs (15 cm²)	
	10 mg/24 hrs (20 cm²)	
	15 mg/24 hrs (30 cm²)	

When Prescribed: Nitro-Dur II is prescribed for relief of angina pectoris (chest pain) which is associated with a decrease in blood flow to the heart muscle.

Precautions and Warnings: Nitro-Dur II should not be given to a patient who is suffering with severe anemia. The strength of this drug is expressed in the area (cm²) and the amount of drug released in 24 hours. Nitro-Dur II is a potent drug. If any of the following side effects occur, contact your physician immediately.

Side Effects and Adverse Reactions: Fainting, weakness, dizziness, headache, vomiting, nausea.

NITROGLYCERIN The generic name for a drug produced by numerous companies in various forms and strengths. Also marketed as:

NITROBID® Marion;
NITROBON® Forest;
NITROL® Kremers-Urban Co.;
NITROSPAN® USV Pharmaceuticals;
NITROSTAT® Parke-Davis & Co.

Dosage Form	Strength	Route
Tablet	0.15 mg	Sublingual (dissolve under tongue)
	0.3 mg	Sublingual
	0.4 mg	Sublingual
	0.6 mg	Sublingual

When Prescribed: Nitroglycerin is prescribed for the relief of attacks of angina pectoris that are often present in various forms of heart disease. This preparation increases the blood flow to the heart muscle.

Precautions and Warnings: Nitroglycerin should be dissolved under the tongue or between the gum and cheek. Do not swallow the tablet. If blurred vision or dryness of mouth occurs, discontinue use and consult your physician.

Side Effects and Adverse Reactions: Blurred vision, dryness of mouth, transient headaches, loss of balance, weakness, heart flutters, fainting.

NITROSTAT® (Parke-Davis and Company)

Generic Name: Nitroglycerin

Dosage Form	Strength	Route
Tablet	0.15 mg	Sublingual (dissolve under tongue)
	0.3 mg	Sublingual
	0.4 mg	Sublingual
	0.6 mg	Sublingual

When Prescribed: Nitrostat is prescribed for the relief of attacks of angina pectoris that are often present in various forms of heart disease. This preparation increases the blood flow to the heart muscle.

Precautions and Warnings: Nitrostat should be dissolved under the tongue or between the gum and cheek. Do not swallow the tablet. If blurred vision or dryness of mouth occurs, discontinue use and consult your physician.

Side Effects and Adverse Reactions: Blurred vision, dryness of mouth, transient headache, loss of balance, weakness, heart flutters, fainting.

NIZORAL® (Janssen Pharmaceutica, Inc.)

Generic Name: Ketoconazole

Dosage Form	Strength	Route
Tablet	200 mg	Oral

When Prescribed: Nizoral is prescribed for the treatment of systemic fungal infections.

Precautions and Warnings: Nizoral should be avoided when the patient is taking antacids and some common cold preparations. Nizoral is associated with severe liver damage which may cause death. If any of the following occur, patient should inform the physician immediately: Fatigue, anorexia, nausea, vomiting, dark urine, or pale stool.

Side Effects and Adverse Reactions: Rash, abdominal pain, nausea, vomiting, diarrhea, headache, enlargement of breasts in men, dizziness, decreased sperm count, photophobia.

NOLVADEX® (ICI Pharma)

Generic Name: Tamoxifen Citrate

Dosage Form	Strength	Route
Tablet	10 mg	Oral

When Prescribed: Nolvadex is prescribed for the treatment of breast cancer in women.

Precautions and Warnings: Fetal damage may occur when taken by pregnant mothers. Do not become pregnant and use barrier, or nonhormonal contraception. Nolvadex should be used with caution in patients with anemia or blood clotting and by nursing mothers.

Side Effects and Adverse Reactions: Are relatively mild and usually easily controlled by regulation of dosage size with hot flashes, nausea, and vomiting occurring most frequently. Less frequently: vaginal bleeding or discharge, menstrual irregularities, and skin rash.

NORDETTE 28® (Wyeth-Ayerst)

Generic Name: Levonorgestrol

Dosage Form	Strength	Route
Tablet	.15 mg/.03 mg	Oral

When Prescribed: Nordette is an oral contraceptive prescribed for purposes of birth control.

Precautions and Warnings: Oral contraceptives are powerful and effective drugs which can have serious side effects including blood clots, strokes, heart attacks, liver tumors, gallbladder disease, and high blood pressure. Safe use of this drug requires a discussion with your physician. A booklet has been prepared to provide you with additional information. Ask your doctor for this booklet. If any of the symptoms listed below are noticed, or anything unusual occurs, consult your physician immediately. Cigarette smoking greatly increases the risk of cardiovascular side effects. Women who use this drug should not smoke.

Side Effects and Adverse Reactions: Nausea, vomiting, abdominal cramps, bloating, bleeding or spotting at times other than during menstruation, change in menstrual flow, pain associated with menstruation, absence of menstruation, temporary infertility after discontinuing treatment, swelling, abnormal darkening of the skin, breast changes, including tenderness, enlargement, and secretion, increase or decrease in body weight, change in vaginal secretions, reduction in amount of breast milk if taken after childbirth, yellowing of skin or eyes, headaches, rash, depression, vaginal infections, cramps, difficulty with contact lenses, uncontrollable

NORGESIC® (Riker Laboratories, Inc.)

Generic Name: Orphenadrine citrate, aspirin, caffeine

Dosage Form	Strength	Route
Tablet	Available in one strength only	Oral

When Prescribed: Norgesic is prescribed for the relief of mild to moderate pain of muscle or skeletal disorders. It is often prescribed for muscle pulls, cramps, sprains. It may also be prescribed to control pain of arthritis, dental procedures, menstruation, or minor surgery.

Precautions and Warnings: Since severe adverse reactions can occur when Norgesic is taken with certain pain relievers such as Darvon, you should only take Norgesic with other medication if your physician directs you to do so. The safe use of Norgesic in pregnant women or children has not been established. This drug may impair your ability to drive or operate machinery.

Side Effects and Adverse Reactions: Rapid heart, irregular heartbeat, inability to urinate, dry mouth, blurred vision, dilation of pupils, eye pressure, weakness, nausea, vomiting, headache, dizziness, constipation, drowsiness, rash, hives, excitation, confusion, hallucinations, lightheadedness, fainting.

Nordette 28-(Continued)

body movements, change in sex drive, change in appetite, nervousness, dizziness, increase of facial hair, loss of scalp hair, itching, skin eruptions.

NORINYL® (Syntex [F.P.], Inc.)

Generic Name: Norethindrone, mestranol

Dosage Form	Strength	Route
Tablet	1/50 21	Oral
	1/50 28	Oral
	1/80 21	Oral
	1/80 28	Oral
	2 mg	

When Prescribed: Norinyl is an oral contraceptive. In the 1/50 and 1/80 forms it is prescribed for birth control only. In the 2 mg form it is prescribed for birth control and menstrual irregularities.

Precautions and Warnings: Oral contraceptives are powerful and effective drugs which can have serious side effects including blood clots, strokes, heart attacks, liver tumors, gall bladder disease, and high blood pressure. Safe use of this drug requires a discussion with your physician. A booklet has been prepared to provide you with additional information. Ask your doctor for this booklet. If any of the symptoms listed below are noticed, or anything unusual occurs, consult your physician immediately. Cigarette smoking increases the risk of cardiovascular side effects. Women who use Norinyl should not smoke.

Side Effects and Adverse Reactions: Nausea, vomiting, abdominal cramps, bloating, bleeding or spotting at times other than during menstruation, change in menstrual flow, pain associated with menstruation, absence of menstruation, temporary infertility after discontinuing treatment, swelling, abnormal darkening of the skin, breast changes including tenderness, enlargement, and secretion, increase or decrease in body weight, change in vaginal secretions, re-

NORMODYNE® (Schering Corporation)

Generic Name: Labetalol hydrochloride

Dosage Form	Strength	Route
Tablet	100 mg	Oral
	200 mg	Oral
	300 mg	Oral

When Prescribed: Normodyne is prescribed for the management of high blood pressure. It can be used with other drugs including diuretics.

Precautions and Warnings: Normodyne should not be used by patients with asthma or heart failure or by patients with a slower heart rate than normal. Don't interrupt or stop Normodyne therapy without informing your physician. During pregnancy and lactation periods, patients should use this drug with caution. Normodyne should be stored at temperatures between 2° and 30° C, or 35.6° and 86° F.

Side Effects and Adverse Reactions: Fatigue, headache, nausea, dizziness, breathing problems, nasal stuffiness, ejaculation failure.

Norinyl-(Continued)

duction in amount of breast milk if taken after birth, yellowing of skin or eyes, headaches, rash, depression, vaginal infections, cramps, difficulty with contact lenses, visual difficulties, uncontrollable body movements, change in sex drive, change in appetite, nervousness, dizziness, increase of facial hair, loss of scalp hair, itching, skin eruptions.

NOROXIN® (Merck Sharp & Dohme)

Generic Name: Norfloxacin, (MSD)

Dosage Form	Strength	Route
Tablet	400 mg	Oral

When Prescribed: Noroxin is a synthetic, antibacterial agent prescribed for the treatment of adults with urinary tract infections caused by susceptible strains of bacteria. Susceptibility should be verified by test.

Precautions and Warnings: Patients with a history of allergic reactions to norfloxacin or the quinolone group of antibiotics should not take Noroxin. Although it is generally well tolerated, pregnant women and children should not take Noroxin. It should be avoided by nursing mothers. Drink sufficient fluids and do not exceed the prescribed daily dosage. Noroxin may impair the physical abilities required for the performance of potentially hazardous tasks such as driving or operating machinery.

Side Effects and Adverse Reactions: Nausea, headache, dizziness, lightheadedness, fatigue, rash, abdominal pain, heartburn, constipation.

NORPRAMINE® (Merrell Dow Pharmaceuticals, Inc.)

Generic Name: Desipramine hydrochloride

Dosage Form	Strength	Route
Tablet	10 mg	Oral
	25 mg	Oral
	50 mg	Oral
	75 mg	Oral
	100 mg	Oral
	150 mg	Oral

When Prescribed: Norpramine is prescribed for relief of symptoms of various types of depression, especially those biochemical in nature.

Precautions and Warnings: If you are suffering with any type of heart disease, thyroid disease, or any problem related to urination and/or seizures, you should inform your physician before starting this therapy. It should be avoided by pregnant women and nursing mothers. It is not recommended for use by children, since safety and effectiveness for children have not been established. Norpramine should not be taken with alcohol, sedatives, tranquilizers, or other sleeping pills. You should not drive or operate machinery after taking this drug.

Side Effects and Adverse Reactions: Hypotension, hypertension, increase in heart rate, change in heart rhythm, anxiety, restlessness, dry mouth, blurred vision, constipation, increase or decrease in libido, breast enlargement in men, impotence, skin rash.

NOVAFED-A® (Merrell Dow Pharmaceuticals, Inc.)

Generic Name: Pseudoephedrine hydrochloride, chlorpheniramine maleate

Dosage Form	Strength	Route
Capsule	Available in one strength only	Oral

When Prescribed: Novafed-A is a combination of antihistamine and decongestant. It is prescribed to provide relief from symptoms associated with the common cold.

Precautions and Warnings: Novafed-A should not be used by patients with high blood pressure or other heart diseases. All antihistamine preparations, including Novafed-A, are not recommended for patients with glaucoma, urinary retention, diabetes, peptic ulcer, or asthmatic attacks.

Side Effects and Adverse Reactions: Increased heart rate, headache, dizziness, nausea, mild sedation, anxiety, sleeping problems, convulsions, change in heart rhythm.

NOVAHISTINE® DH (Dow Pharmaceuticals)

Generic Name: Codeine phosphate, chlorpheniramine maleate, alcohol, pseudoephidrine hydrochloride

Dosage Form	Strength	Route
Liquid	Available in one strength only	Oral

When Prescribed: Novahistine DH is prescribed for relief from cough and nasal congestion, due to colds or other respiratory infections. It can also be prescribed for relief of congestion in ears.

Precautions and Warnings: Novahistine may interact with other drugs you are taking. This drug may be habit forming. The codeine in Novahistine may potentiate the effects of alcohol, pain relievers, sleeping pills and sedatives. If drowsiness occurs, do not drive or operate machinery.

Side Effects and Adverse Reactions: Nausea, vomiting, constipation, dizziness, sedation, heart flutters, fear, anxiety, tenseness, restlessness, shaking, weakness, pale skin, difficulty in breathing, urinary problems, insomnia, hallucinations, convulsions, itching.

NUCOFED® (Beecham Laboratories)

Generic Name: Codeine phosphate, pseudoephedrine hydrochloride, sucrose (only in syrup), alcohol (only in expectorant)

Dosage Form	Strength	Route
Capsule	Available in one strength only	Oral
Syrup	Same as above	Oral
Expectorant	Same as above	Oral
Pediatric Expectorant	Same as above	Oral

When Prescribed: Nucofed is prescribed for relief from coughing and congestion associated with upper respiratory tract infections and related conditions such as common cold, bronchitis, influenza, and sinus inflammation.

Precautions and Warnings: Persons with persistent cough, asthma and other lung diseases, high blood pressure, heart disease, diabetes, or thyroid disease should not take this product except under the advice and supervision of a physician. It may cause or aggravate constipation. This product is not recommended for children who are taking some other drugs. Nucofed should not be given to pregnant women or nursing mothers. One of the ingredients is codeine phosphate, which may be habit forming.

Side Effects and Adverse Reactions: Nervousness, restlessness, trouble sleeping, drowsiness, headache, nausea, vomiting, constipation, trouble breathing, increase in sweating, weakness, change in heart rate.

NYSTATIN The generic name for a drug produced by numerous companies in different dosage forms. Some of these are:
MYCOSTATIN® Squibb;
NILSTAT® Lederle;
NYSTEX® Savage.

Dosage Form	Strength	Route
Cream	100,000 units/gm	Topical (apply directly to affected area)
Ointment	100,000 units/gm	Topical
Powder	100,000 units/gm	Topical
Suspension	100,000 units/ml	Oral
Tablet	500,000 units	Oral
Vaginal Tablet	100,000 units	Intra-vaginal

When Prescribed: Nystatin preparations are prescribed for the treatment of infection caused by *Candida* (a fungus found in nature). It is prescribed for local, oral, and intravaginal use, depending on the site of infection.

Precautions and Warnings: If a patient is using the topical preparation, there is possibility of hypersensitivity reaction. In this case, withdraw the treatment immediately. When using intravaginally, the patient should be warned against interruption or discontinuation of medication even during menstruation and even though symptomatic relief may occur within a few days.

Side Effects and Adverse Reactions: When used locally, if irritation occurs, discontinue the medication. Large oral doses may cause diarrhea, gastrointestinal distress, nausea, and vomiting. When sensitization or irritation occurs on intravaginal use of this drug, it should be reported to the physician immediately.

OGEN® (Abbott Laboratories)

Generic Name: Estropipate

Dosage Form	Strength	Route
Tablet	.625 mg	Oral
	1.5 mg	Oral
	2.5 mg	Oral
	5 mg	Oral
Cream	1.5 mg/gm	Intra-vaginal

When Prescribed: Ogen is prescribed for the treatment of estrogen deficiency associated with certain specific conditions.

Precautions and Warnings: Ogen and other estrogens have been reported to increase the risk of cancer of the inner layer of the uterine wall. Ogen should not be used during pregnancy. Estrogen preparations are associated with some severe side effects. If any of the following occur, contact your physician immediately.

Side Effects and Adverse Reactions: Breast tenderness, withdrawal bleeding, vaginal candidiasis, painful menstruation, breakthrough bleeding, spotting, change in menstrual flow, premenstrual-like syndrome, enlargement of breasts, vomiting, nausea, abdominal cramps, skin rash, loss of scalp hair, mental depression, dizziness, headache, increase or decrease in weight, change in sexual function.

OMNIPEN® (Wyeth Laboratories)

Generic Name: Ampicillin

Dosage Form	Strength	Route
Capsule	250 mg	Oral
	500 mg	Oral
Suspension	125 mg/5 ml	Oral
	250 mg/5 ml	Oral

When Prescribed: Omnipen is a semisynthetic penicillin that is effective in a wide variety of infections.

Precautions and Warnings: Omnipen should not be taken by people who are allergic to penicillin. The use of any penicillin should be discontinued and your physician notified if any of the side effects listed below appear.

Side Effects and Adverse Reactions: Nausea, vomiting, chest or stomach pains, diarrhea, changes in color/texture of tongue and oral mucous membranes, skin rash, hives, chills, fever, swelling, pain in joints, fainting, super-infection by nonsusceptible organisms, anemia, abnormal bruising, indigestion, darkening of urine.

ORGANIDIN® (Wallace Laboratories)

Generic Name: Iodinated glycerol

Dosage Form	Strength	Route
Drops	5%	Oral
Elixir	1.2%	Oral
Tablet	30 mg	Oral

When Prescribed: Organidin is prescribed as an expectorant in respiratory tract conditions such as bronchitis, asthma, chronic inflammation of sinuses, or after surgery to help prevent pulmonary collapse.

Precautions and Warnings: Patients sensitive to iodide should not take Organidin. It also causes a flare-up of adolescent acne in some individuals. Organidin should not be taken by pregnant women, nursing mothers, or newborns.

Side Effects and Adverse Reactions: Gastric irritation, rash, thyroid gland enlargement.

ORNADE® SPANSULES® (Modified Formula) (Smith Kline and French Laboratories)

Generic Name: Chlorpheniramine maleate, phenylpropanolamine hydrochloride

Dosage Form	Strength	Route
Capsule (time release)	Available in one strength only	Oral

When Prescribed: Ornade is prescribed for the relief of sneezing, running nose, watery eyes, and nasal congestion associated with the common cold, sinus infections, hay fever, and allergies.

Precautions and Warnings: Ornade is not intended for use in children under 6. Patients should not drive or operate machinery while taking this drug. Ornade should not be taken with alcohol, tranquilizers, sleeping pills, or sedatives.

Side Effects and Adverse Reactions: Drowsiness; excessive dryness of nose, throat, or mouth; nervousness; insomnia; nausea; vomiting; heartburn; diarrhea; rash; dizziness; weakness; tightness of chest; pain in chest or abdomen; irregular heartbeat; headache; tremors; lack of coordination; painful or difficult urination; anemia; convulsions; changes in blood pressure; loss of appetite; constipation; visual disturbances; acne; swollen glands.

ORTHO-NOVUM® (Ortho Pharmaceuticals)

Generic Name: Norethindrone, mestranol

Dosage Form	Strength		Route
Tablet	1/35	21	Oral
	1/35	28	Oral
	1/50	21	Oral
	1/50	28	Oral
	1/80	21	Oral
	1/80	28	Oral
	2 mg		Oral
	10 mg		Oral

When Prescribed: Ortho-Novum is an oral contraceptive. In the 1/50 and 1/80 forms, it is prescribed for birth control only. In the 2 mg and 10 mg forms, it is prescribed for birth control and menstrual irregularities.

Precautions and Warnings: Oral contraceptives are powerful and effective drugs which can cause serious side effects including blood clots (which may lead to strokes, heart attacks), liver tumors, gall bladder disease and high blood pressure. Safe use of this drug requires a discussion with your physician. A booklet has been prepared to provide you with additional information. Ask your doctor for this booklet. If any of the symptoms listed below are noticed or anything unusual occurs, consult your physician immediately. Cigarette smoking increases the risk of cardiovascular side effects. Women taking Ortho-Novum should not smoke.

Side Effects and Adverse Reactions: Nausea, vomiting, abdominal cramps, bloating, bleeding or spotting at times other than during menstruation, change in menstrual flow, pain associated with

ORUDIS® (Wyeth-Ayerst)

Generic Name: Ketoprofen

Dosage Form	Strength	Route
Capsules	25 mg	Oral
	50 mg	Oral
	75 mg	Oral

When Prescribed: Orudis is prescribed for the treatment of rheumatoid arthritis, osteoarthritis, mild-to-moderate pain, and painful menstruation.

Precautions and Warnings: Orudis can induce gastrointestinal bleeding, ulceration and perforation. Patients with kidney problems should use Orudis with caution. Pregnant women, and nursing mothers should avoid Orudis. It is not recommended for children.

Side Effects and Adverse Reactions: Peptic ulcer, GI bleeding, nausea, heartburn, abdominal pain, diarrhea, gas, anorexia, vomiting, headache, dizziness, swelling of the mouth, visual disturbances, rash, urinary tract irritation, kidney problems, increased appetite, dry mouth, belching, rectal bleeding, bloody stool, amnesia, confusion, impotence, migraine, vertigo, conjunctivitis, eye pain, hearing impairment, sweating, skin rash and discoloration, hypertension, heart palpitations, congestive heart failure, anemia, thirst, weight gain or loss, liver problems, muscular pain, labored and shortness of breath.

OVCON-35 28® (Mead Johnson)

Generic Name: Norethindrone, ethinyl estradiol

Dosage Form	Strength	Route
Tablet	.4 mg/35 mcg	Oral

When Prescribed: Ovcon-35 28 is a 28-day regimen of oral contraception.

Precautions and Warnings: Women who take oral contraceptives should not smoke. Cigarette smoking while taking oral contraceptives greatly increases the risk of heart attack. Oral contraceptives are potent drugs. Safe use of Ovcon-35 28 requires a thorough discussion with your doctor. A booklet has been prepared for your use. Ask your physician for a copy of this booklet. Maintain regular physical examinations and follow-up. If any of the symptoms listed below are noticed, or anything unusual occurs, consult your physician immediately.

Side Effects and Adverse Reactions: Nausea, vomiting, abdominal cramps, blotting, bleeding, or spotting at times other than during menstruation, change in menstrual flow, pain associated with menstruation, absence of menstruation, temporary infertility after discontinuing treatment, swelling, abnormal darkening of the skin, breast changes including tenderness, enlargement, and secretion, increase or decrease in body weight, change in vaginal secretions, reduction in amount of breast milk if taken after birth, yellowing of skin or eyes, headaches, rash, depression, vaginal infections, cramps, difficulty with contact lenses, visual dif-

OVRAL® (Wyeth Laboratories)

Generic Name: Norgestrel, ethinyl estradiol

Dosage Form	Strength	Route
Tablet	Available in one strength only	Oral

When Prescribed: Ovral is an oral contraceptive. Like other contraceptives it is a combination of estrogen and progesterone.

Precautions and Warnings: Oral contraceptives are powerful and effective drugs which can have serious side effects including blood clots, strokes, heart attacks, liver tumors, gall bladder disease and high blood pressure. Safe use of this drug requires a discussion with your physician. A booklet has been prepared to provide you with additional information. Ask your doctor for this booklet. If any of the symptoms listed below are noticed or anything unusual occurs, consult your physician immediately. Cigarette smoking increases the risk of cardiovascular side effects. Women who take Ovral should not smoke.

Side Effects and Adverse Reactions: Nausea, vomiting, abdominal cramps, bloating, bleeding or spotting at times other than during menstruation, change in menstrual flow, pain associated with menstruation, absence of menstruation, temporary infertility after discontinuing treatment, swelling, abnormal darkening of the skin, breast changes including tenderness, enlargement, and secretion, increase or decrease in body weight, changes in vaginal secretions, reduction in amount of breast milk if

Ortho-Novum-(Continued)

menstruation, absence of menstruation, temporary infertility after discontinuing treatment, swelling, abnormal darkening of the skin, breast changes including tenderness, enlargement, and secretion, increase or decrease in body weight, changes in vaginal secretions, reduction in amount of breast milk if taken after childbirth, yellowing of skin or eyes, headaches, rash, depression, vaginal infections, cramps, difficulty with contact lenses, visual difficulties, uncontrollable body movements, change in sex drive, change in appetite, dizziness, increase of facial hair, loss of scalp hair, itching, skin eruptions, changes in personality such as nervousness.

Ovcon-35 28-(Continued)

ficulties, uncontrollable body movements, change in sex drive, change in appetite, nervousness, dizziness, increase of facial hair, loss of scalp hair, itching, skin eruptions.

Ovral-(Continued)

taken after childbirth, yellowing of skin or eyes, headaches, rash, depression, vaginal infections, cramps, difficulty with contact lenses, visual difficulties, uncontrollable body movements, change in sex drive, change in appetite, nervousness, dizziness, increase of facial hair, loss of scalp hair, itching, skin eruptions.

137

PAMELOR® (Sandoz Pharmaceuticals)

Generic Name: Nortriptyline

Dosage Form	Strength	Route
Capsules	10 mg	Oral
	25 mg	Oral
	50 mg	Oral
	75 mg	Oral
Solution	10 mg	Oral

When Prescribed: Pamelor is an antidepressant prescribed to relieve the symptoms of depression.

Precautions and Warnings: Do not use Pamelor with a monoamine oxidase (MAO) inhibitor, if you are allergic to the drug, or during recovery from a heart attack. Patients with heart disease should take Pamelor only under close medical supervision. It should be used with great caution in patients who have glaucoma, a history of urinary retention, seizures, hyperthyroidism, or who are taking thyroid medication. Patients should not drive or operate machinery while taking Pamelor. Alcohol combined with Pamelor is dangerous in patients with histories of emotional disturbances or suicidal attempts. The safe use of Pamelor during pregnancy, nursing, and in children has not been established. The use of Pamelor may induce schizophrenic episodes in those patients. Overactive, agitated patients may experience increased anxiety. The manic-depressive patient may experience manic episodes. Because of the potential for suicide, dosages should be closely monitored.

Side Effects and Adverse Reactions: Heart disease, stroke, confusion, hallucinations, disorientation, delusions, anxiety, panic, insomnia, nightmares,

PARAFON FORTE® (McNeil Laboratories, Inc.)

Generic Name: Chlorzoxazone, acetaminophen

Dosage Form	Strength	Route
Tablet	Available in one strength only	Oral

When Prescribed: Parafon Forte is prescribed for the relief of pain and stiffness of muscle and bone disorders. It is often prescribed for chronic muscle spasm.

Precautions and Warnings: The safe use of this drug in pregnancy has not been established.

Side Effects and Adverse Reactions: Gastrointestinal disturbances, drowsiness, dizziness, light-headedness, depression, stimulation, rashes, discoloration of urine, skin eruptions, hives.

Pamelor-(Continued)

worsened psychosis, numbness, tingling, tremors, dry mouth, blurred vision, constipation, urinary retention, dialation of urinary tract, breast and testicular swelling, impotence, jaundice, flushing, perspiration, altered weight, fatigue, headache.

PARLODEL® (Sandoz Pharmaceuticals)

Generic Name: Bromocriptine mesylate

Dosage Form	Strength	Route
Tablet	2½ mg	Oral
Capsule	5 mg	Oral

When Prescribed: Parlodel is prescribed to treat high prolactin levels in the blood, because of which a woman may suffer excessive discharge of milk, failure of menstruation, and infertility.

Precautions and Warnings: If you are sensitive to any ergot alkaloids, inform your physician. Patients using Parlodel can suffer from hypotension (decrease in blood pressure). If pregnancy occurs during Parlodel administration, treatment should be discontinued immediately. Since Parlodel prevents lactation, it should not be given to nursing mothers. Safety and efficacy of Parlodel have not been established for children under 15. Safety and efficacy of Parlodel have not been established for patients with kidney and liver disease. Some of the drugs for psychological disorders should not be used with Parlodel (ask your physician/pharmacist). Any other medications which decrease blood pressure should be used with caution with Parlodel.

Side Effects and Adverse Reactions: Nausea, headache, dizziness, fatigue, abdominal cramps, vomiting, lightheadedness, nasal congestion, constipation, diarrhea.

PCE/ERYTHROMYCIN PARTICLES IN TABLETS® (Abbott)

Generic Name: Erythromycin

Dosage Form	Strength	Route
Tablet	333 mg	Oral

When Prescribed: PCE is an antibiotic prescribed to treat a wide range of infections caused by susceptible strains of bacteria in diseases including respiratory tract infections, pneumonia, whooping cough, PID (pelvic inflammatory disease) and syphillis.

Precautions and Warnings: PCE should not be taken by patients with a known allergic reaction to erythromycin. Liver disorder may occur with or without jaundice. Prolonged use may induce superinfection, thus requiring more appropriate therapy.

Side Effects and Adverse Reactions: Gastrointestinal, dosed-related side effects occur most frequently: vomiting, abdominal pain, diarrhea, anorexia, liver dysfunction, skin rash.

PEDIAZOLE® (Ross Laboratories)

Generic Name: Erythromycin
ethylsuccinate, sulfisoxazole acetyl

Dosage Form	Strength	Route
Liquid	Available in one strength only	Oral

When Prescribed: Pediazole is prescribed for the treatment of ear infections in children.

Precautions and Warnings: This drug is not recommended for infants less than 2 months of age.

Side Effects and Adverse Reactions: Abdominal cramping and discomfort, nausea, vomiting, diarrhea, rash, hives, itching, pain in the joints, loss of appetite, headache, depression, convulsion, loss of balance, hallucinations, ringing in the ears, insomnia, fever, chills, urinary problems.

PENICILLIN V POTASSIUM 400,000 UNITS The generic name of a drug produced by numerous companies in various forms and strengths. Also marketed as:
PEN-VEE K®
V-CILLIN K® Eli Lilly and Co.;
VEETIDS® Squibb.

Generic Name: Penicillin V potassium

Dosage Form	Strength	Route
Tablet	125 mg 200,000 units	Oral
	250 mg 400,000 units	Oral
	500 mg 800,000 units	Oral
Liquid	125 mg 200,000 units	Oral
	250 mg 400,000 units	Oral

When Prescribed: Penicillin V potassium is prescribed for the treatment of mild to moderately severe infections by organisms which are susceptible to this type of penicillin. There are different types of penicillin, each of which is effective in different infections. Your physician determines which type is the proper one to use in your particular case.

Precautions and Warnings: Serious hypersensitivity (allergic) reactions can occur in susceptible individuals. For maximum absorption, dosage should be given on an empty stomach. If any of the symptoms listed below occurs, consult your physician immediately.

Side Effects and Adverse Reactions: Nausea, vomiting, heartburn, diarrhea, changes in color/texture of oral membranes, skin rash, skin eruptions, hives, chills, fever, swelling, pain in joints, fainting, difficult breathing, anemia, sore mouth, superinfection by nonsusceptible organisms.

PEN-VEE® K (Wyeth Laboratories)

Generic Name: Penicillin V potassium

Dosage Form	Strength	Route
Tablet	125 mg 200,000 units	Oral
	250 mg 400,000 units	Oral
	500 mg 800,000 units	Oral
Liquid	125 mg 200,000 units	Oral
	250 mg 400,000 units	Oral

When Prescribed: Pen-Vee K is prescribed for the treatment of mild to moderately severe infections by organisms which are susceptible to this type of penicillin. There are different types of penicillin, each of which is effective in different infections. Your physician determines which type is the proper one to use in your particular case.

Precautions and Warnings: Serious hypersensitivity (allergic) reactions can occur in susceptible individuals. For maximum absorption, dosage should be given on an empty stomach. If any of the symptoms listed below occurs, consult your physician immediately.

Side Effects and Adverse Reactions: Nausea, vomiting, heartburn, diarrhea, changes in color/texture of oral membranes, skin rash, skin eruptions, hives, chills, fever, swelling, pain in joints, fainting, difficult breathing, anemia, sore mouth, superinfection by non-susceptible organisms.

PEPCID® (Merck, Sharp, & Dohme)

Generic Name: Famotidine

Dosage Form	Strength	Route
Tablet	20 mg	Oral
	40 mg	Oral
Suspension	40 mg	Oral

When Prescribed: Pepcid is used in short-term and maintenance treatment of duodenal ulcers and in short-term treatment of gastric ulcers.

Precautions and Warnings: Relief of symptoms does not rule out the presence of malignancy. Reduce dosage for patients with kidney disease. Nursing mothers should carefully consider use of the drug. Its safety and effectiveness in children has not been established.

Side Effects and Adverse Reactions: Headache, dizziness, constipation and diarrhea.

PERCOCET-5® (Endo Laboratories, Inc.)

Generic Name: Oxycodone hydrochloride, acetaminophen

Dosage Form	Strength	Route
Tablet	Available in one strength only	Oral

When Prescribed: Percocet-5 is prescribed for the relief of moderate to moderately severe pain.

Precautions and Warnings: This drug can possibly be physically addictive. Psychological dependence and tolerance (a larger dose is necessary to produce the same effect) can also occur. Patients taking this drug may become drowsy. If so, they should not drive or operate dangerous machinery. Percocet should not be taken with alcohol, tranquilizers, sleeping pills or sedatives unless specifically directed by your physician. The safe use of this drug in pregnant women and children has not been established.

Side Effects and Adverse Reactions: Lightheadedness, dizziness, sedation, nausea, vomiting, mood changes, constipation, itching, skin rash.

PERCODAN® (Endo Laboratories, Inc.)

Generic Name: Oxycodone hydrochloride, oxycodone terephthalate, aspirin, phenacetin, caffeine

Dosage Form	Strength	Route
Tablet	Full strength	Oral
Tablet (Perdocan demi)	Half strength	Oral

When Prescribed: Percodan is prescribed for the relief of moderate to moderately severe pain. Percodan contains a narcotic pain reliever and therefore is prescribed only when weaker medication is deemed ineffective.

Precautions and Warnings: Percodan can produce drug dependence and therefore has the potential for abuse. Physical and/or psychological dependence can occur. Patients using this drug should not drive or use dangerous machinery. Percodan should not be taken with alcohol, tranquilizers, sedatives or sleeping pills. This drug is not recommended for use during pregnancy nor for use by children.

Side Effects and Adverse Reactions: Lightheadedness, dizziness, sedation, nausea, vomiting, altered states of mood, constipation and itching.

PERIACTIN® (Merck Sharp and Dohme)

Generic Name: Cyproheptadine hydrochloride

Dosage Form	Strength	Route
Tablet	4 mg	Oral
Syrup	2 mg/5 ml	Oral

When Prescribed: Periactin is an antihistamine prescribed for nasal congestion, hay fever and allergies; for swollen eyes due to pollen and food allergies; for mild skin allergies manifested as rash or hives; for allergic reactions from blood transfusions; and for various other allergic reactions.

Precautions and Warnings: Patients using this drug should not drive or operate dangerous machinery. Alcohol, tranquilizers, sedatives and sleeping pills should not be used with this drug. Mothers should not nurse while taking this drug.

Side Effects and Adverse Reactions: Drowsiness, dry mouth, dizziness, jitteriness, faintness, dryness of the mucous membranes, headache, nausea, rash, swelling, agitation, confusion, hallucinations, difficulty urinating, fatigue, restlessness, tremors, irritability, tingling or numbness in hands, excessive perspiration, chills, insomnia, euphoria, loss of appetite, vomiting, diarrhea, constipation, irregular heartbeat, tightness of chest, wheezing, rash, hives, visual disturbances, menstrual irregularities.

PERSANTINE® (Boehringer Ingelheim Ltd.)

Generic Name: Dipyridamole

Dosage Form	Strength	Route
Tablet	25 mg	Oral
	50 mg	Oral
	75 mg	Oral

When Prescribed: Persantine is prescribed to increase the blood flow in surgical patients following cardiac valve replacement.

Precautions and Warnings: Persantine should be used with caution in patients with hypotension. It should be used in pregnant women only if clearly needed and should be used with caution in nursing mothers. The safety and effectiveness of this drug in children below 12 years has not been established.

Side Effects and Adverse Reactions: Dizziness, abdominal distress, headache, rash.

143

PHENAPHEN® with CODEINE
(A. H. Robins Company)

Generic Name: Codeine phosphate, acetaminophen

Dosage Form	Strength	Route
Capsule	No. 2	Oral
	No. 3	Oral
	No. 4	Oral

When Prescribed: Phenaphen is prescribed for the relief of pain.

Precautions and Warnings: This preparation may be habit forming with prolonged use or overuse. If drowsiness occurs, you should not drive or operate machinery. Should not be taken with alcohol, tranquilizers, sedatives or sleeping pills. The safe use of Phenaphen with codeine during pregnancy has not been established.

Side Effects and Adverse Reactions: Drowsiness, nausea, constipation, lightheadedness, dizziness, euphoria, uneasiness, sedation, nausea and vomiting.

PHENERGAN® SYRUP PLAIN (Wyeth Laboratories)

Generic Name: Promethazine hydrochloride, alcohol

Dosage Form	Strength	Route
Liquid	Available in one strength only	Oral

When Prescribed: Phenergan syrup is prescribed for nasal and chest congestion due to hay fever, allergies, or colds.

Precautions and Warnings: This drug contains a mild sedative. Patients using Phenergan should not drive or operate machinery. This drug should not be taken with alcohol, tranquilizers, sedatives, or sleeping pills.

Side Effects and Adverse Reactions: Dryness of mouth, blurred vision, dizziness, changes in blood pressure, increased skin sensitivity to sunlight.

PHENERGAN® with CODEINE (Wyeth Laboratories)

Generic Name: Promethazine, alcohol, codeine phosphate

Dosage Form	Strength	Route
Liquid	Available in one strength only	Oral

When Prescribed: Phenergan with Codeine is prescribed for the same reasons as Phenergan Syrup. In addition, the former contains codeine, which will suppress coughs that may accompany such conditions.

Precautions and Warnings: In addition to the precautions and warnings for Phenergan Syrup, this drug may be habit forming.

Side Effects and Adverse Reactions: In addition to the side effects possible with Phenergan Expectorant, this drug may cause constipation or nausea.

PHENERGAN® VC EXPECTORANT (Wyeth Laboratories)

Generic Name: Promethazine hydrochloride, phenylephrine hydrochloride, alcohol

Dosage Form	Strength	Route
Liquid	Available in one strength only	Oral

When Prescribed: Phenergan VC Expectorant is prescribed for the same reasons as Phenergan Syrup. In addition, it contains phenylephrine hydrochloride, which will help dry mucous membranes.

Precautions and Warnings: This drug contains a mild sedative. Patients using Phenergan should not drive or operate machinery. This drug should not be taken with alcohol, tranquilizers, sedatives, or sleeping pills.

Side Effects and Adverse Reactions: Dryness of mouth, blurred vision, dizziness, changes in blood pressure, increased skin sensitivity to sunlight.

PHENERGAN® VC with CODEINE
(Wyeth Laboratories)

Generic Name: Promethazine hydrochloride, phenylephrine hydrochloride, alcohol, codeine phosphate

Dosage Form	Strength	Route
Liquid	Available in one strength only	Oral

When Prescribed: Phenergan VC with Codeine is prescribed for nasal and chest congestion due to hay fever, allergies, or colds. This drug contains codeine which will help suppress coughs.

Precautions and Warnings: Codeine may be habit forming. If drowsiness occurs, you should not drive or operate dangerous machinery. Phenergan VC with Codeine should not be taken with alcohol, sleeping pills, sedatives, or tranquilizers.

Side Effects and Adverse Reactions: Dryness of mouth, blurred vision, dizziness, increased sensitivity to sunlight, constipation, nausea.

PHENOBARBITAL
The generic name for a drug produced by numerous companies in various forms and strengths.

Generic Name: Phenobarbital

Dosage Form	Strength	Route
Tablet	15 mg	Oral
	30 mg	Oral
	60 mg	Oral
	100 mg	Oral
Extended-release capsule	8 mg	Oral
	16 mg	Oral
	32 mg	Oral
	65 mg	Oral
	100 mg	Oral

When Prescribed: Phenobarbital is a sedative and sleep-inducing drug which is prescribed for a variety of reasons, among which are anxiety, tension, restlessness, hyperactivity, insomnia and epilepsy.

Precautions and Warnings: Phenobarbital may be habit forming. Patients taking this drug should not drive or operate machinery. Phenobarbital should not be taken with alcohol, sedatives, sleeping pills or tranquilizers. The safe use of phenobarbital in pregnancy has not been established.

Side Effects and Adverse Reactions: Drowsiness, hangover, dizziness, loss of balance, headache, nausea, skin eruptions, rash, hives, excitement, confusion, depression, lethargy, vomiting.

POLARAMINE® (Schering Corporation)

Generic Name: Dexchlorpheniramine maleate (alcohol in syrup)

Dosage Form	Strength	Route
Syrup	2 mg/5 ml	Oral
Tablets	2 mg	Oral
	4 mg	Oral
Repetabs® (timed release)	6 mg	Oral

When Prescribed: Polaramine is prescribed for relief of symptoms from hay fever, nasal congestion, allergic skin rash, itching, poison ivy or oak, insect bites, drug reactions, asthma, and other disorders that are treatable with antihistamines.

Precautions and Warnings: If drowsiness occurs, you should not drive or operate dangerous machinery.

Side Effects and Adverse Reactions: Drowsiness, dizziness, nausea, restlessness, dry mouth, weakness, loss of appetite, headache, nervousness, frequent urination, heartburn, double vision, sweating, urinary difficulties, skin irritation.

POLY-VI-FLOR® (Mead Johnson Laboratories)

Generic Name: Multiple vitamins plus fluoride

Dosage Form	Strength	Route
Tablet	1 mg F	Oral
	0.5 mg F	Oral
Drops	0.25 mg F	Oral
	0.5 mg F	Oral

When Prescribed: This preparation is prescribed for children to prevent vitamin deficiencies and to supply fluoride for prevention of tooth decay in areas where the fluoride content of the water is low.

Precautions and Warnings: Poly-Vi-Flor should only be used in areas where the fluoride content of the drinking water is below 0.7 parts per million. Do not give more than prescribed. Keep out of reach of children.

Side Effects and Adverse Reactions: Overuse can lead to fluoride poisoning. Rash may develop in children allergic to this preparation.

POTASSIUM CHLORIDE The generic
name for a drug produced by numerous
companies and marketed in various forms
and strengths. Also marketed as:
K-LOR®, Abbott;
K-LYTE/CL®, Mead Johnson Pharmaceutical;
KAOCHLOR®, Warren-Teed;
KAY CIEL®, Berlex;
KEFF®, Lemmon;
KLOR-CON®, Upsher-Smith;
KLORVESS®, Dorsey;
KOLYUM®, Pennwalt;
RUM-K®, Fleming;
SLOW-K®, Ciba.

Generic Name: Potassium chloride

Dosage Form	Strength	Route

Available in various forms and strengths to be taken orally.

When Prescribed: Potassium chloride is prescribed to replace potassium, an essential salt, in patients who are deficient in potassium. Potassium deficiency can result from the use of drugs that control blood pressure, among other reasons.

Precautions and Warnings: Potassium-containing drugs are often upsetting to the stomach. For this reason many of the drugs will be in the form of a tablet or powder which should be dissolved completely before taking. Gastrointestinal upset can be reduced if the drug is taken with meals. If the drug is in a liquid form, it should be sipped slowly over a five-to-ten-minute period.

Side Effects and Adverse Reactions: Nausea, vomiting, diarrhea, abdominal discomfort.

PRED® FORTE (Allergan Pharmaceuticals, Inc.)

Generic Name: Predisolone acetate

Dosage Form	Strength	Route
Suspension (eye drops)	Available in one strength only	Eye Drops

When Prescribed: Pred Forte is prescribed for inflammatory conditions of the eye that are responsive to steroids.

Precautions and Warnings: Pred Forte should not be used in certain types of eye infections. Long-term use of Pred Forte may cause a fungal infection of the eye. Pred Forte should be used with caution by patients with a history of herpes simplex infections.

Side Effects and Adverse Reactions: Optic nerve damage, defect in visual field, secondary eye infections.

PREDNISONE

PREDNISONE The generic name of a drug produced by numerous companies in various strengths. Also marketed as:
DELTASONE® Upjohn;
DELTRA® Merck Sharp and Dohme;
METICORTEN® Schering.

Dosage Form	Strength	Route
Tablet	2.5 mg	Oral
	5.0 mg	Oral
	10 mg	Oral
	20 mg	Oral
	50 mg	Oral

When Prescribed: Prednisone is a hormone which is primarily noted for its potent antiinflammatory effect. It is prescribed for endocrine disorders, arthritis, collagen disease, skin diseases, allergic reactions, eye diseases, respiratory diseases, blood disorders, cancer of the blood, water retention, and various other diseases.

Precautions and Warnings: Prednisone is a potent drug which should be used only under close supervision of a physician. Patients should not receive smallpox immunization or other inoculations while on Prednisone therapy.

Side Effects and Adverse Reactions: Water retention, heart failure, muscle weakness, loss of muscle, bone fractures, ulcer, abdominal distention, wounds that heal slowly, thin fragile skin, skin eruptions, increased sweating, convulsions, dizziness, headache, menstrual irregularities, masculinization of females, suppression of growth in children, decreased ability to withstand stress, intensification of existing diabetes, cataracts, glaucoma.

PREMARIN

PREMARIN® (Ayerst Laboratories)

Generic Name: Conjugated estrogens

Dosage Form	Strength	Route
Tablet	0.3 mg	Oral
	0.625 mg	Oral
	1.25 mg	Oral
	2.5 mg	Oral

Note: Also available in vaginal cream.

When Prescribed: Estrogens are secreted by the ovary and are responsible for the development and maintenance of the female reproductive system. Premarin is often prescribed for estrogen replacement for deficiencies caused by menopause, and other conditions where ovarian output of estrogen is diminished. Premarin may be prescribed for abnormal uterine bleeding due to hormonal imbalance. It is prescribed for the prevention of breast enlargement after childbirth and sometimes in the treatment of breast cancers. In males, it may be used in the treatment of cancer of the prostate.

Precautions and Warnings: Premarin is not recommended for use during pregnancy. Premarin should be used only under close supervision by your physician. Increased instances of dangerous side effects including cancer and blood clots have been reported with estrogen compounds. Should not be used for "prolonged" periods of time.

Side Effects and Adverse Reactions: Nausea, vomiting, loss of appetite, abdominal cramps, bloating, bleeding or spotting at times other than menstruation, breast tenderness and enlargement, reduction in milk production when given

PRINIVIL® (Merck Sharp & Dohme)

Generic Name: Lisinopril (MSD)

Dosage Form	Strength	Route
Tablets	5 mg	Oral
	10 mg	Oral
	20 mg	Oral
	40 mg	Oral

When Prescribed: Prinivil is prescribed for hypertension and can be used alone or in combination with other high-blood-pressure medication.

Precautions and Warnings: Those patients who have shown an allergic reaction to any of Prinivil's components and patients with a history of angioedema (swelling) as a result of a prior treatment with medication in this class of drugs should not take Prinivil. Although Prinivil is generally well tolerated, swelling of the face has occurred in some patients. When facial swelling occurs, Prinivil should be immediately discontinued and the patient closely observed until the swelling subsides. If the larynx, glottis, and tongue are involved, emergency therapy should be given at once. Patients with congestive heart failure and others susceptible to kidney failure should use Prinivil with caution.

Side Effects and Adverse Reactions: Dizziness, headache, fatigue, diarrhea, upper respiratory symptoms, cough, nausea, hypotension, rash, orthostatic effects, weakness, chest pain, vomiting, indigestion, shortness of breath, labored breath, numbness of extremities, impotence, muscle cramps, back pain, nasal congestion, decreased sex drive, vertigo.

PROCAN SR® (Parke-Davis and Company)

Generic Name: Procainamide hydrochloride

Dosage Form	Strength	Route
Tablet	250 mg	Oral
	500 mg	Oral
	750 mg	Oral
	1000 mg	Oral

When Prescribed: Procan SR is prescribed to treat abnormal rhythm of the heart.

Precautions and Warnings: If a patient using Procan SR experiences aches and malaise (feelings of general discomfort), he should contact the physician immediately. Do not crush or chew the tablet. If you miss a dose and remember within one hour or so, take it as soon as possible. Then go back to your regular dosing schedule. Do not take double doses.

Side Effects and Adverse Reactions: Malaise and aches; soreness of the mouth, throat, and gums; unexplained fever; skin rash; unusual bleeding or bruising; symptoms that resemble arthritis or upper respiratory tract infections.

Premarin-(Continued)

after childbirth, in males loss of sex drive and development of breasts, water retention, aggravation of migraine headaches, headache, allergic rash, dizziness, abnormal weight changes, inability to wear contact lenses, beard growth in females, loss of hair.

PROCARDIA® (Pfizer Laboratories Division)

Generic Name: Nifedipine

Dosage Form	Strength	Route
Capsule	10 mg	Oral
Capsule	20 mg	Oral

When Prescribed: Procardia is prescribed to help prevent attacks of angina that often occur in patients with heart disorders.

Precautions and Warnings: The safe use of this drug in pregnancy has not been established.

Side Effects and Adverse Reactions: Dizziness, lightheadedness, giddiness, flushing, heat sensation, headache, weakness, nausea, heartburn, muscle cramps, tremor, swelling, nervousness, mood changes, heart flutters, breathing difficulties, cough, wheezing, nasal congestion, sore throat, fainting, increased anginal pain, chest congestion, diarrhea, constipation, gas, pain or stiffness in the joints, shakiness, jitteriness, sleep disturbances, blurred vision, loss of balance, itching, rash, hives, sweating, chills, fever, sexual difficulties.

PROLIXIN® (E. R. Squibb & Sons)

Generic Name: Fluphenazine hydrochloride

Dosage Form	Strength	Route
Tablets	1 mg	Oral
	2.5 mg	Oral
	5 mg	Oral
	10 mg	Oral

When Prescribed: Prolixin is prescribed for management of certain emotional disorders. It has *not* been shown effective in management of behavior abnormalities in mentally retarded people.

Precautions and Warnings: Prolixin tablets (except 1 mg) contain FD&C yellow No. 5 (a dye), which may cause an allergic-type reaction including asthma. It is frequently seen in patients who also have aspirin hypersensitivity. Safe use of this drug during pregnancy and for children has not been established. This drug should not be stopped abruptly. If any soreness of mouth, gum, or throat or any symptoms of upper respiratory tract infection occurs, therapy should be discontinued.

Side Effects and Adverse Reactions: Tremors; jerky movements; involuntary movements of tongue; face, mouth, or jaw; insomnia; restlessness; anxiety; mood alteration; lethargy; headache; confusion; loss of appetite; salivation; constipation; anemia; weight change; abnormal lactation; enlargement of breasts in males; menstrual irregularities; false results on pregnancy tests; impotency in males; increased libido in females.

PROPINE® (Allergan Pharmaceuticals Inc.)

Generic Name: Dipivefrin hydrochloride

Dosage Form	Strength	Route
Ophthalmic Eye Solution	Available in one strength only	Eye Drop

When Prescribed: Propine is prescribed to control internal pressure of the eye in open-angle glaucoma.

Precautions and Warnings: Propine should not be used in narrow-angle glaucoma. This drug should be used in pregnancy only if it is clearly needed. It should be used with caution by nursing mothers. Its safety for children has not been established.

Side Effects and Adverse Reactions: Increase in heart rate, change in heartbeat, increase in blood pressure, burning and stinging of eye.

PROPRANOLOL HYDROCHLORIDE

The generic name for a drug produced by numerous companies.

Dosage Form	Strength	Route
Tablet	10 mg	Oral
	20 mg	Oral
	40 mg	Oral
	80 mg	Oral

When Prescribed: Propranolol hydrochloride is a potent drug which is prescribed for various heart conditions such as angina pectoris. It is intended to help the heart beat at a normal rhythm. It is also used to control symptoms of certain tumors of the nervous system, for high blood pressure, and for migraine headache.

Precautions and Warnings: Patients using this drug should be closely monitored and should not abruptly discontinue the drug after long-term use. If any of the side effects listed below appear, your physician should be contacted immediately.

Side Effects and Adverse Reactions: Slow heartbeat, heart failure, low blood pressure, numbness or tingling of the hands, lightheadedness, insomnia, lassitude, weakness, fatigue, mental depression, visual disturbances, hallucinations, disorientation, memory loss, changes in emotions, nausea, vomiting, heartburn, cramps, diarrhea, constipation, rash, fever, sore throat, respiratory distress, anemia, loss of hair.

PROTOSTAT® (Ortho Pharmaceutical Corporation)

Generic Name: Metronidazole

Dosage Form	Strength	Route
Tablet	250 mg	Oral
	500 mg	Oral

When Prescribed: Protostat is prescribed for treatment of certain infections (trichomoniasis) of the genital tract in both males and females. It is also prescribed for treatment of dysentery (amebic dysentery) and liver abscess caused by amoebas.

Precautions and Warnings: Alcoholic beverages should not be consumed during Protostat therapy, because abdominal cramps, vomiting, and flushing may occur. The drug is not recommended for use during early pregnancy. It should not be used by nursing mothers.

Side Effects and Adverse Reactions: Nausea, headache, loss of appetite, cramps, diarrhea, unpleasant metallic taste, constipation, dizziness, numbness, joint pains, rash, hives, weakness, frequent urination, nasal congestion, superinfection by nonsusceptible organisms.

PROVENTIL® (Schering Corporation)

Generic Name: Albuterol

Dosage Form	Strength	Route
Inhaler	Available in one strength only	Oral inhalation
Tablet	2 mg	Oral
	4 mg	

When Prescribed: Proventil is prescribed for the relief of breathing difficulty associated with some diseases of the lung.

Precautions and Warnings: Do not use more often than prescribed. The safe use of this drug in pregnant women has not been established. Proventil is not recommended for nursing mothers or children under 12 years of age.

Side Effects and Adverse Reactions: Heart flutters, rapid heartbeat, tremor, nausea, dizziness, heartburn, nervousness, pain in chest or arm, vomiting, loss of balance, stimulation, insomnia, headache, unusual taste, dryness or irritation of the nose or throat.

PROVERA® (The Upjohn Company)

Generic Name: Medroxyprogesterone acetate

Dosage Form	Strength	Route
Tablet	2.5 mg	Oral
	10 mg	Oral

When Prescribed: Provera is a form of progesterone which is prescribed for the induction of menstruation in women for whom menstruation is irregular or absent, and for women (who are not pregnant) suffering from uterine bleeding or painful menstruation.

Precautions and Warnings: The use of progesterone substances such as Provera can result in a number of adverse side effects or reactions, some of which can be fatal. If you notice any side effects while taking this drug, consult your physician at once.

Side Effects and Adverse Reactions: Breast tenderness, abnormal milk production, adverse effects on child if taken during pregnancy, hives, rash, skin eruptions, increase in facial hair, blood clots, abnormal menstrual bleeding, water retention, weight change, yellowing of skin or eyes, itching, mental depression, increase in blood pressure, changes in sex drive, changes in appetite, headache, nervousness, dizziness, fatigue, backache, loss of scalp hair.

PROZAC® (Lilly)

Generic Name: Fluoxetine hydrochloride

Dosage Form	Strength	Route
Pulvules (Capsules)	20 mg	Oral

When Prescribed: Prozac is an antidepressant and is prescribed for the treatment of depression.

Precautions and Warnings: This preparation may cause drowsiness. Therefore, driving motor vehicles or operating dangerous machinery is discouraged while on Prozac. It should be used with caution by patients with liver and kidney disease or a history of seizures. It should not be used during nor within at least 14 days following the administration of monoamine oxidase (MAO) inhibitors and use of MAO inhibitors should be delayed for five weeks following use of Prozac. Notify your physician immediately if you develop a rash or hives, drink alcohol, plan to take other prescription or over-the-counter drugs, become pregnant, or breast feed. Physical or psychological dependence on Prozac has not been sufficiently studied.

Side Effects and Adverse Reactions: Impairment of thinking, judgment, and motor skills; anxiety, nervousness, drowsiness, dizziness, lightheadedness, headaches, insomnia, nausea, diarrhea, tremor, fatigue, dry mouth, anorexia, weight loss, indigestion, constipation, stomach pain, vomiting, gas, sweating, rash, increased appetite, abnormal dreams, decreased sex drive, bronchitis.

PYRIDIUM® (Parke-Davis and Company)

Generic Name: Phenazopyridine
hydrochloride

Dosage Form	Strength	Route
Tablet	100 mg	Oral
	200 mg	Oral

When Prescribed: Pyridium is prescribed for the symptomatic relief of pain, burning, urgency, frequency and other discomforts accompanying urination. These symptoms may result from infection, trauma, surgery, examination procedures or other factors which cause irritation of the lower urinary tract.

Precautions and Warnings: The reddish-orange discoloration of the urine is due to the drug and is normal.

Side Effects and Adverse Reactions: Gastrointestinal disturbances.

QUESTRAN LIGHT® (Bristol-Myers)

Generic Name: Cholestyramine Resin

Dosage Form	Strength	Route
Powder	4 g	Oral

When Prescribed: Questran Light is prescribed as an adjunct to reduce serum cholesterol when diet alone has not adequately worked.

Precautions and Warnings: Do not take Questran Light in its dry form, always mix with water. Patients experiencing bile duct obstructions should not take Questran. Before beginning therapy with cholestyramine, hypothyroidism, diabetes, liver disease, and other diseases contributing to elevated serum cholesterol should be looked for and treated. A downward trend should occur within the first month of Questran therapy. Make every effort to avoid severe constipation while taking cholestyramine. Inform physician of pregnancy or nursing. Since Questran may inhibit their action other drugs should be taken one hour before or four to six hours after ingestion of Questran. The effect of long-term Questran administration in children and infants is not known.

Side Effects and Adverse Reactions: Constipation, nausea, vomiting, diarrhea, heartburn, anorexia, bleeding due to vitamin K deficiency.

QUINAGLUTE® (Berlex Laboratories)

Generic Name: Quinidine gluconate

Dosage Form	Strength	Route
Tablets	324 mg	Oral

When Prescribed: Quinaglute is prescribed to increase the contractibility of the heart muscle. It may also be used to treat irregular rhythm of the heart.

Precautions and Warnings: If you are using any other drug, your physician should be informed before you start on Quinaglute. There are possibilities of hypersensitivity reactions with this drug, especially during the first weeks after starting therapy. If you notice abnormalities, inform your physician immediately.

Side Effects and Adverse Reactions: Nausea, headache, ringing in the ears, disturbances in vision, abdominal pain, diarrhea, changes in heart rate, decrease in blood pressure, anemia, blurred vision, night blindness, reduced visual field, rash.

QUINAMM® (Merrell-National Laboratories, Inc.)

Generic Name: Quinine sulfate

Dosage Form	Strength	Route
Tablet	Available in one strength only	Oral

When Prescribed: Quinamm is prescribed for the relief of leg muscle cramps that occur in bed.

Precautions and Warnings: This drug should not be taken by pregnant women.

Side Effects and Adverse Reactions: Easy bruising, visual problems, ringing in the ears, loss of hearing, loss of balance, headache, nausea, vomiting, fever, apprehension, restlessness, confusion, fainting, rash, hives, itching, flushing of skin, sweating, swelling of the face, heartburn, difficulty breathing, pain in chest or arm.

REGLAN® (A. H. Robins Company)

Generic Name: Metoclopramide hydrochloride

Dosage Form	Strength	Route
Tablet	10 mg	Oral

When Prescribed: Reglan is prescribed for the relief of gastrointestinal symptoms suffered by some diabetics.

Precautions and Warnings: Report any abnormal effects, including abnormal body or facial movements, to your physician.

Side Effects and Adverse Reactions: Restlessness, drowsiness, fatigue, lassitude, insomnia, headache, dizziness, nausea, bowel disturbance.

RESTORIL® (Sandoz Pharmaceuticals)

Generic Name: Temazepam

Dosage Form	Strength	Route
Capsule	15 mg 30 mg	Oral

When Prescribed: Restoril is prescribed to help induce sleep in people who have difficulty sleeping, including difficulty falling asleep, frequent awakenings during the night, and/or early-morning awakenings.

Precautions and Warnings: Restoril should not be combined with alcohol, sedatives, tranquilizers or other sleeping pills. Persons using this drug should not drive or operate dangerous machinery. Restoril should not be taken during pregnancy. Sleep may be disturbed for a few nights after Restoril has been discontinued. The safety of this drug in children under the age of 18 has not been established.

Side Effects and Adverse Reactions: Drowsiness, dizziness, lethargy, confusion, euphoria, relaxed feeling, weakness, loss of appetite, diarrhea, tremors, loss of balance, lack of concentration, falling down, heart flutters, hallucinations, abnormal eye movements, excitement, stimulation, hyperactivity.

RETIN-A® (Ortho Pharmaceutical Corporation)

Generic Name: Tretinoin

Dosage Form	Strength	Route
Gel	0.025% 0.010%	Topical (apply to the affected skin)
Cream	0.050% 0.100%	Topical
Liquid	0.050%	Topical

When Prescribed: Retin-A is prescribed for certain kinds of acne.

Precautions and Warnings: Patients using this preparation should attempt to minimize their exposure to sunlight or to ultraviolet lamps. If exposure cannot be avoided, the use of a sunscreen over the treated areas is suggested.

Side Effects and Adverse Reactions: Reddening of the skin, blisters, swelling of skin, crusting of skin, change in skin color, hypersensitivity to sunlight.

RITALIN® (Ciba Pharmaceutical Company)

Generic Name: Methylphenidate hydrochloride

Dosage Form	Strength	Route
Tablet	5 mg	Oral
	10 mg	Oral
	20 mg	Oral

When Prescribed: This drug is prescribed for a syndrome called attention deficit disorder (previously known as minimal brain dysfunction in children), for narcolepsy, a disorder of the sleep mechanism in which uncontrolled or abnormal sleep occurs, and also to treat mild depression or senile behavior.

Precautions and Warnings: Chronically abusive use of this drug can lead to psychological dependence with varying degrees of abnormal behavior. The safe use of this drug in pregnancy has not been established.

Side Effects and Adverse Reactions: Nervousness, insomnia, skin rash, hives, fever, pain in joints, skin eruptions, loss of appetite, nausea, dizziness, blood pressure and pulse changes (both up and down), abdominal pain, weight loss, anemia, scalp hair loss, abnormal movements or tremors, headache, irregular heartbeat.

ROBAXIN® (A. H. Robins Company)

Generic Name: Methocarbamol

Dosage Form	Strength	Route
Tablet	500 mg	Oral
	750 mg	Oral

When Prescribed: Robaxin is prescribed for the relief of discomfort associated with muscle-skeletal disorders. The relaxation brought about by Robaxin is thought to be due to a general nervous system depression.

Precautions and Warnings: Robaxin is not recommended for use during pregnancy or for nursing mothers. Safety and effectiveness of Robaxin in children under the age of 12 has not been established. If drowsiness occurs, you should not drive or operate dangerous machinery.

Side Effects and Adverse Reactions: Lightheadedness, dizziness, drowsiness, nausea, rash, eye irritation, visual disturbances, nasal congestion, blurred vision, headache, fever.

ROBITUSSIN A-C® (A. H. Robins Company)

Generic Name: Guaifenesin, codeine phosphate, alcohol

Dosage Form	Strength	Route
Liquid	Available in one strength only	Oral

When Prescribed: Robitussin A-C is prescribed to control cough that can accompany various disorders.

Precautions and Warnings: Robitussin A-C contains codeine which may be habit forming.

Side Effects and Adverse Reactions: Nausea, gastrointestinal upset, constipation, drowsiness.

ROBITUSSIN-DAC® (A. H. Robins Company)

Generic Name: Guaifenesin, pseudoephedrine hydrochloride, codeine phosphate

Dosage Form	Strength	Route
Liquid	Available in one strength only	Oral

When Prescribed: Robitussin-DAC is prescribed for the temporary relief of cough and nasal congestion that may occur with the common cold or because of inhalation of irritants.

Precautions and Warnings: Use this product with caution if prescribed for children under 2 years or children taking another drug. Caution should be taken in administering this drug to patients with high blood pressure, heart disease, shortness of breath, or diabetes. Do not exceed recommended dosage. At higher doses, nervousness, dizziness, or sleepiness may occur.

Side Effects and Adverse Reactions: Agitation, dizziness, insomnia, nausea.

RONDEC-DM® (Ross Laboratories)

Generic Name: Carbinoxamine maleate, pseudoephedrine hydrochloride, dextromethorphan hydrobromide, alcohol

Dosage Form	Strength	Route
Syrup	Available in one strength only	Oral
Drops	Available in one strength only	Oral

When Prescribed: Rondec-DM is prescribed for the relief of symptoms of the common cold, nose irritation, bronchitis and related respiratory conditions.

Precautions and Warnings: The safe use of this drug in pregnancy has not been established. Patients should avoid alcohol and other nervous system depressants. If drowsiness occurs, you should not drive or operate dangerous machinery.

Side Effects and Adverse Reactions: Sedation, dizziness, double vision, vomiting, dry mouth, headache, nervousness, nausea, loss of appetite, heartburn, weakness, urinary difficulties, excitability, convulsions, depression, heart flutters, breathing difficulties, rapid heartbeat, hallucinations, tremors, nervousness, insomnia, weakness, pale skin.

RU-TUSS® (Boots Pharmaceutical, Inc.)

Generic Name: Phenylephrine hydrochloride, phenylpropanolamine hydrochloride, chlorpheniramine maleate, hyoscyamine sulfate, atropine sulfate, scopolamine hydrobromide.

Dosage Form	Strength	Route
Tablet	Available in one strength only	Oral

When Prescribed: Ru-Tuss is prescribed to relieve the symptoms of irritations of the sinuses, nose, and upper respiratory tract.

Precautions and Warnings: If drowsiness occurs, you should not drive or operate dangerous machinery. Ru-Tuss should not be taken with alcohol, sleeping pills, tranquilizers or sedatives unless indicated by your physician. This preparation is not recommended for children under 12 years old.

Side Effects and Adverse Reactions: Rash, itching, hives, drowsiness, lack of energy, giddiness, dryness of the mucous membranes, tightness of the chest, thickening of bronchial secretions, urinary problems, heart flutters, rapid heartbeat, faintness, dizziness, ringing in the ears, headache, loss of coordination, visual disturbances, loss of appetite, nausea, vomiting, diarrhea, constipation, heartburn, irritability, nervousness, insomnia.

RUFEN® (Boots Pharmaceuticals, Inc.)

Generic Name: Ibuprofen

Dosage Form	Strength	Route
Tablet	400 mg	Oral
	600 mg	Oral

When Prescribed: Rufen is prescribed to relieve pain and inflammation of arthritis. Rufen is as effective as aspirin for long-term management of pain and inflammation but usually is better tolerated in terms of stomach upset and irritation. Rufen is also prescribed for pains and cramps related to menstruation.

Precautions and Warnings: Rufen is not recommended during pregnancy or nursing or for patients who are suffering with peptic ulcers. The use of aspirin with Rufen may reduce the effectiveness of the drug. Rufen should not be used by patients who exhibit bronchospastic reactivity to aspirin.

Side Effects and Adverse Reactions: Nausea, chest pains, heartburn, diarrhea, constipation, gastric pain, vomiting, indigestion, bloating, gas, dizziness, headache, nervousness, rash, ringing in the ears, decreased appetite, depression, insomnia, visual disturbances, nightmares, fever, itching.

RYNATAN® (Wallace Laboratories)

Generic Name: Phenylephrine tannate

Dosage Form	Strength	Route
Tablet	Available in one strength only	Oral
Suspension	Available in one strength only	Oral

When Prescribed: Rynatan is prescribed for symptomatic relief of nasal congestion associated with the common cold, allergy, and other respiratory tract conditions.

Precautions and Warnings: Rynatan should be used with caution by patients suffering from hypertension, diabetes, thyroid problems, glaucoma, or enlarged prostates. This drug should not be used with alcohol, tranquilizers, or sleeping pills.

Side Effects and Adverse Reactions: Drowsiness; sedation; dryness of mouth, nose, and throat; gastrointestinal effects.

SELDANE® (Merrell Dow Pharmaceutical Inc.)

Generic Name: Terfenadine

Dosage Form	Strength	Route
Tablet	60 mg	Oral

When Prescribed: Seldane is prescribed for relief of symptoms associated with seasonal allergy such as sneezing, runny nose, and lacrimation.

Precautions and Warnings: Seldane should not be given to pregnant women, nursing mothers, or children under 12. Drowsiness is possible with Seldane; therefore, patients should refrain from activities requiring mental alertness.

Side Effects and Adverse Reactions: Drowsiness, headache, fatigue, dizziness, nervousness, weakness, appetite increase, dry mouth, dry nose, dry throat.

SELSUN® (Abbott Laboratories)

Generic Name: Selenium sulfide, detergent

Dosage Form	Strength	Route
Liquid (shampoo)	Available in one strength only	Apply to scalp

When Prescribed: Selsun is a shampoo prescribed for the treatment of common dandruff and flaking of scalp.

Precautions and Warnings: Oiliness of the hair may increase following use of the lotion. Yellow or orange discoloration of gray or white hair may occur but can usually be avoided by careful rinsing. Safe use on infants has not been established.

Side Effects and Adverse Reactions: Increased sensitivity of scalp or adjacent areas.

SEPTRA® (Burroughs Wellcome Company)

Generic Name: Trimethoprim, sulfamethoxazole

Dosage Form	Strength	Route
Tablet	Regular strength	Oral
Tablet	Double strength	Oral
Liquid	Available in one strength only	Oral

When Prescribed: Septra is a combination of drugs prescribed for the treatment of certain types of urinary tract infections and for certain other types of bacterial infections.

Precautions and Warnings: Septra is not recommended during pregnancy or for nursing mothers. If any of the side effects or adverse reactions listed below appear, consult your physician.

Side Effects and Adverse Reactions: Rash, sore throat, stomach upset, nausea, vomiting, abdominal pains, diarrhea, yellowing of skin, headache, body aches, depression, convulsions, hallucinations, ringing in the ears, dizziness, loss of balance, insomnia, apathy, fatigue, weakness, nervousness, fever, chills, urinary difficulties.

SER-AP-ES® (Ciba Pharmaceutical Company)

Generic Name: Reserpine, hydralazine hydrochloride, hydrochlorothiazide

Dosage Form	Strength	Route
Tablet	Available in one strength only	Oral

When Prescribed: Ser-ap-es is prescribed for the control of high blood pressure. This drug is prescribed only after your physician has determined that the fixed combination of drugs in this preparation is correct for you.

Precautions and Warnings: Ser-ap-es is a potent drug which should be used only under close supervision of your physician. The safe use of this drug in pregnancy has not been established.

Side Effects and Adverse Reactions: Oversecretion of stomach acid, nausea, vomiting, loss of appetite, diarrhea, chest pains, heart flutters, slowing of heart, drowsiness, depression, nervousness, anxiety, nightmares, tremors, dull sensations, deafness, eye disorders, nasal congestion, itching, rash, hives, skin eruptions, painful or difficult urination, muscle aches, weight gain, breast enlargement, lactation, breast development in males, increased heart rate, numbness or tingling of skin, yellow skin or eyes, hepatitis, constipation, yellow appearance of objects, increased sensitivity to sunlight, anemia, changes in blood pressure, fever, chills, diminished sex drive.

SERAX® (Wyeth Laboratories)

Generic Name: Oxazepam

Dosage Form	Strength	Route
Capsule	10 mg	Oral
	15 mg	Oral
	30 mg	Oral
Tablet	15 mg	Oral

When Prescribed: Serax is prescribed for a wide variety of problems to provide relief from tension, anxiety and related symptoms. It is used in a wide variety of physical and/or emotional disorders, also in skeletal muscle spasm, and to treat symptoms of acute alcohol withdrawal. This product has been found to be particularly useful in older patients.

Precautions and Warnings: The use of Serax during pregnancy should almost always be avoided. Excessive use of this drug can cause a dependency. If drowsiness occurs, patients should not drive or operate dangerous machinery. Serax can lower tolerance to alcohol.

Side Effects and Adverse Reactions: Drowsiness, dizziness, loss of balance, headache, fainting, rashes, nausea, slurred speech, shaking, change in sex drive, anxiety, visual disturbances, nightmares, excitation and confusion, disorientation, fever, euphoria.

SILVADENE® CREAM (Marion Laboratories, Inc.)

Generic Name: Silver sulfadiazine

Dosage Form	Strength	Route
Cream	1%	Topical (apply directly to affected area)

When Prescribed: Silvadene Cream is prescribed as an adjunct therapy for prevention and treatment of wound sepsis in patients with burns.

Precautions and Warnings: Silvadene Cream should not be used at term pregnancy, on premature infants, and/or on newborn infants during the first month of life. Safe use of Silvadene Cream during pregnancy has not been established. If any problems occur in urination, inform your physician. Drink plenty of water when using this cream.

Side Effects and Adverse Effects: Rash, burning, itching.

SINEMET® (Merck Sharp and Dohme)

Generic Name: Levodopa, carbidopa

Dosage Form	Strength	Route
Tablet	10/100 25/100 25/250	Oral

When Prescribed: Sinemet is prescribed for the treatment of the symptoms of Parkinson's disease.

Precautions and Warnings: The safe use of this drug in pregnancy has not been established. Sinemet should not be taken by nursing mothers or children under 18 years of age.

Side Effects and Adverse Reactions: Nausea, heart flutters, abnormal movements, slow movements, loss of appetite, dizziness, vomiting, personality changes, blood in stool or vomit, black stool or vomit.

SINEQUAN® (Pfizer Laboratories Division)

Generic Name: Doxepin HCl

Dosage Form	Strength	Route
Capsule	10 mg	Oral
	25 mg	Oral
	50 mg	Oral
	75 mg	Oral
	100 mg	Oral
	150 mg	Oral
Concentrated liquid	Available in one strength only	Oral

When Prescribed: Sinequan is prescribed for relief from anxiety, tension, depression, sleep disturbances, guilt, lack of energy, fear, apprehension and worry resulting from both physical and psychological disorders.

Precautions and Warnings: Sinequan may interact with other drugs. Be sure your physician is advised of all drugs you are taking. This drug is not recommended for children under the age of 12. If drowsiness occurs, you should not drive or operate dangerous machinery. Tolerance to alcohol may be lowered.

Side Effects and Adverse Reactions: Dry mouth, blurred vision, constipation, urinary difficulties, drowsiness, confusion, disorientation, hallucinations, numbness, tingling of skin, dizziness, loss of balance, rash, nausea, vomiting, indigestion, taste disturbances, diarrhea, loss of appetite, altered sex drive, impotence, ringing in the ears, weight gain, sweating, chills, fatigue, weakness, headache, loss of hair, development of breasts in males, enlargement of breasts in females, rapid heartbeat, increased sensitivity to sunlight.

SINGLET® (Dow Pharmaceuticals)

Generic Name: Phenylephrine hydrochloride, chlorpheniramine maleate, acetaminophen

Dosage Form	Strength	Route
Tablet	Available in one strength only	Oral

When Prescribed: Singlet is prescribed to reduce congestion, secretions, pain and fever resulting from colds, hay fever, sinus problems, flu, and other conditions.

Precautions and Warnings: This drug may have dangerous interactions with other drugs you may be taking. Singlet is not recommended for use by nursing mothers. If drowsiness occurs, do not drive or operate dangerous machinery. Not recommended for children under 12.

Side Effects and Adverse Reactions: Drowsiness, restlessness, dry mouth, dizziness, weakness, loss of appetite, nausea, headache, nervousness, urinary problems, heartburn, double vision, skin irritations, nausea, vomiting, anxiety, tenseness, tremors, loss of color, respiratory difficulties, sleeplessness, convulsions, heart flutters.

SLO-BID® (William H. Rorer, Inc.)

Generic Name: Theophylline

Dosage Form	Strength	Route
Capsule	50 mg	Oral
	100 mg	Oral
	200 mg	Oral
	300 mg	Oral

When Prescribed: Slo-Bid is prescribed for relief and/or prevention of symptoms of asthma and reversible bronchospasms associated with chronic bronchitis and emphysema.

Precautions and Warnings: If you are a smoker, you might need more doses of this drug compared to nonsmokers. Your physician should be informed if symptoms occur repeatedly, especially near the end of a dosing interval. It should be avoided by pregnant women and nursing mothers. Safety and effectiveness for children under 6 have not been established.

Side Effects and Adverse Reactions: Nausea, vomiting, gastric pain, diarrhea, headache, irritability, restlessness, insomnia, convulsions, palpitations, increase in heart rate, change in heart rhythm, increase in blood sugar level, rash.

SLO-PHYLLIN® (William H. Rorer, Inc.)

Generic Name: Theophylline anhydrous

Dosage Form	Strength	Route
Syrup	80 mg/15 ml	Oral
Tablets	100 mg	Oral
	200 mg	
Capsule (time release)	60 mg	Oral
	125 mg	
	250 mg	

When Prescribed: Slo-Phyllin is prescribed for the relief and/or prevention of asthma and breathing difficulties associated with chronic bronchitis or emphysema.

Precautions and Warnings: The safe use of this drug in pregnancy has not been established.

Side Effects and Adverse Reactions: Nausea, vomiting, heartburn, blood in vomit, diarrhea, headache, irritability, restlessness, insomnia, overactive reflexes, muscle twitches, convulsions, heart flutters, rapid heartbeat, flushing, low blood pressure, rapid breathing, frequent urination.

SLOW-K® (Ciba Pharmaceutical Company)

Generic Name: Potassium chloride

Dosage Form	Strength	Route
Tablet	600 mg	Oral

When Prescribed: Slow-K is a preparation formulated to provide a controlled rate or release of potassium chloride in patients whose level of potassium is low. It is often prescribed for patients who are taking certain cardiovascular or high blood pressure drugs (diuretics) that tend to deplete the body of potassium. Because Slow-K can cause ulcers and bleeding, other forms of potassium supplementation are usually prescribed. Slow-K is usually prescribed only in individuals who cannot or will not take these other forms of medication.

Precautions and Warnings: Frequent determinations of potassium levels are necessary while taking this preparation.

Side Effects and Adverse Reactions: Nausea, vomiting, abdominal discomfort, diarrhea, changes in heartbeat, skin rash.

SODIUM SULAMYD® (Schering Corporation)

Generic Name: Sulfacetamide sodium

Dosage Form	Strength	Route
Ophthalamic	30%	Intraocular
solution	10%	(in the eye)

When Prescribed: Sodium sulamyd is prescribed for the treatment of a number of different eye infections.

Precautions and Warnings: These preparations should be stored in a cool place. On long standing, the solutions will darken in color and should be discarded.

Side Effects and Adverse Reactions: Transient stinging or burning of the eye.

SOMA® (Wallace Laboratories)

Generic Name: Carisoprodol

Dosage Form	Strength	Route
Tablet	350 mg	Oral

When Prescribed: Soma is prescribed for relief of discomfort associated with acute, painful musculoskeletal conditions.

Precautions and Warnings: Soma should not be taken by patients who are allergic to meprobamate. Safe use of this drug in pregnancy or by nursing mothers has not been established. Soma is not recommended for children under 12. Soma should not be taken with alcohol, sedatives, tranquilizers, or sleeping pills. Patients taking this drug should not drive or operate machinery. A psychological dependence on Soma can occur.

Side Effects and Adverse Reactions: If any of the following occur with the use of Soma, contact your physician: fever, weakness, dizziness, wheezing, lightheadedness—these signs may precede anaphylactic shock. Other side effects are nausea, vomiting, increase in heart rate, skin rash.

SOMA® COMPOUND (Wallace Laboratories)

Generic Name: Carisoprodol, aspirin

Dosage Form	Strength	Route
Tablet	Available in one strength only	Oral

When Prescribed: Soma Compound combines a muscle relaxant and a pain reliever. It is prescribed for the relief of pain and stiffness in muscles and joints resulting from injury or a chronic problem such as arthritis.

Precautions and Warnings: This drug may impair your mental and/or physical abilities. Patients using this drug should not drive or operate machinery. Soma Compound should not be taken with alcohol, sedatives, tranquilizers, or sleeping pills. The safe use of Soma Compound in pregnancy has not been established. Not recommended for use by nursing mothers or children under 12.

Side Effects and Adverse Reactions: Drowsiness, lightheadedness, dizziness, itching, nervousness, flutters of the heart, weakness, loss of balance, agitation, euphoria, confusion, disorientation, gastrointestinal disturbances, insomnia, frequent urination, headache, fainting, skin rash, burning eyes.

SOMA® COMPOUND with CO-DEINE (Wallace Laboratories)

Generic Name: Carisoprodol, aspirin, codeine phosphate

Dosage Form	Strength	Route
Tablet	Available in one strength only	Oral

When Prescribed: Soma Compound with Codeine is a combination of a muscle relaxant, aspirin, and codeine phosphate. It is prescribed for relief of pain and muscular spasm.

Precautions and Warnings: Soma Compound with Codeine may impair mental and/or physical abilities to drive and operate machinery. Patients with ulcers and other gastrointestinal problems should not use this drug. It should be given to pregnant women only if needed. It should not be given to nursing mothers and children under 12 years of age. If the first dose of Soma Compound with Codeine causes extreme weakness, dizziness, walking abnormality, temporary loss of vision, agitation, euphoria, confusion, or disorientation, the drug should be discontinued.

Side Effects and Adverse Reactions: Dizziness, vertigo, ataxia, tremor, agitation, irritation, headache, depressive reactions, insomnia.

STELAZINE® (Smith Kline and French Laboratories)

Generic Name: Trifluoperazine hydrochloride

Dosage Form	Strength	Route
Tablet	1 mg	Oral
	2 mg	Oral
	5 mg	Oral
	10 mg	Oral

When Prescribed: Stelazine is a potent drug prescribed for the management of certain mental disorders or for the control of the excessive anxiety, tension and agitation seen with emotional or physical disorders.

Precautions and Warnings: Stelazine may impair mental and/or physical abilities, especially during the first few days of therapy. Patients using this drug should not drive or operate machinery. Should not be taken with sedatives, alcohol, tranquilizers or sleeping pills.

Side Effects and Adverse Reactions: Drowsiness, dizziness, skin reactions, rash, dry mouth, insomnia, absence of menstruation, fatigue, muscular weakness, loss of appetite, lactation, blurred vision, tremors, jerky movements, muscle spasms, difficulty swallowing, abnormal facial expressions or movements, anemia, yellowing of skin or eyes, sexual disorders, skin eruptions, eye problems, increased severity of angina in some patients.

STUARTNATAL 1+1® (Stuart Pharmaceuticals)

Generic Name: Multiple vitamins and minerals

Dosage Form	Strength	Route
Tablet	Available in one strength only	Oral

When Prescribed: Stuartnatal 1+1 is prescribed as a vitamin and mineral supplement for pregnant women and nursing mothers.

Precautions and Warnings: Do not exceed recommended dosage.

Side Effects and Adverse Reactions: This drug is well tolerated. No side effects or adverse reactions are listed.

SULTRIN® (Ortho Pharmaceutical Corp.)

Generic Name: Sulfathiazole, sulfacetamide, sulfabenzamide

Dosage Form	Strength	Route
Cream	Available in one strength only	Intravaginal
Vaginal tablet	Available in one strength only	Intravaginal

When Prescribed: Sultrin is prescribed for the treatment of vaginal infections. It may also be prescribed to treat vaginal odor that results from radiation therapy.

Precautions and warnings: If relief is not obtained in 6 to 10 days, consult your physician again.

Side Effects and Adverse Reactions: This drug is well tolerated.

SUMYCIN® (E. R. Squibb & Sons)

Generic Name: Tetracycline hydrochloride

Dosage Form	Strength	Route
Capsule	250 mg	Oral
	500 mg	Oral
Tablet	250 mg	Oral
	500 mg	Oral
Syrup	125 mg/5 cc	Oral

When Prescribed: Sumycin is an effective antibiotic prescribed for many different types of infection. It is often used in place of penicillin in patients who are allergic to penicillin.

Precautions and Warnings: Sumycin should not be taken by people overly sensitive to tetracycline. If any of the side effects listed below occur, consult your physician immediately. Not recommended for pregnant women, infants or children under the age of 8.

Side Effects and Adverse Reactions: Exaggerated sunburn, super-infection by nonsusceptible organisms, loss of appetite, nausea, vomiting, diarrhea, inflammation of the tongue, difficulty swallowing, stomach pains, inflammation of the bowel and genital region, skin rash, hives, swelling, fainting.

SYMMETREL® (DuPont Pharmaceuticals)

Generic Name: Amantadine hydrochloride

Dosage Form	Strength	Route
Capsule	Available in one strength only	Oral

When Prescribed: Symmetrel is prescribed for treatment of Parkinson's disease. It is also prescribed to prevent and treat respiratory tract illness caused by certain strains of virus.

Precautions and Warnings: Patients with a long history of epilepsy or other seizures should be observed closely for possible increased seizure activity. Symmetrel should not be discontinued abruptly. Patients receiving Symmetrel who note blurring of vision should be cautioned against driving or working in situations where alertness is important.

Side Effects and Adverse Reactions: Depression, heart failure, hypotension, psychosis, urinary retention, hallucinations, confusion, anxiety, anorexia, nausea, dry mouth, headache.

SYNALAR® (Syntex Laboratories, Inc.)

Generic Name: Fluocinolone acetonide

Dosage Form	Strength	Route
Cream	0.01%	Topical (Apply directly to affected area)
	0.025%	
Ointment	0.025%	Topical
Solution	0.01%	Topical

When Prescribed: Synalar is a synthetic form of a hormone normally produced in your body. It is prescribed to reduce inflammation and swelling in certain skin disorders.

Precautions and Warnings: Synalar is applied locally and is well tolerated. However, if any irritation develops, consult your physician. Synalar is not for use in the eye. This drug should not be used for prolonged periods of time or in large amounts by pregnant women.

Side Effects and Adverse Reactions: Burning, itching, irritation, dryness, infected hair follicles, acne, loss of pigment, excessive hair growth, skin destruction.

SYNALGOS-DC® (Ives Laboratories, Inc.)

Generic Name: Dihydrocodeine bitartrate, aspirin, caffeine

Dosage Form	Strength	Route
Capsule	Available in one strength only	Oral

When Prescribed: Synalgos-DC is prescribed for the relief of moderate to moderately severe pain in situations where your physician wishes to add a mild sedative effect. This preparation contains a narcotic similar to codeine in addition to a mild sedative, and weaker pain relievers.

Precautions and Warnings: Because it contains a substance similar to codeine, Synalgos-DC may be habit forming. If drowsiness occurs, you should not drive or operate dangerous machinery. The safe use of this drug in pregnant patients has not been established. This drug is not recommended for children.

Side Effects and Adverse Reactions: Lightheadedness, dizziness, drowsiness, sedation, nausea, vomiting, constipation, itching, skin reactions.

SYNTHROID® (Flint Laboratories)

Generic Name: Sodium levothyroxine

Dosage Form	Strength	Route
Tablet	.025 mg	Oral
	.050 mg	Oral
	.1 mg	Oral
	.15 mg	Oral
	.2 mg	Oral
	.3 mg	Oral

When Prescribed: Synthroid is synthetically produced thyroid gland hormone. Synthroid is prescribed when the body produces insufficient thyroid hormone. This can be due to a variety of reasons, some of which are surgery, disease, birth defect and radiation.

Precautions and Warnings: Synthroid therapy should be closely regulated by your physician.

Side Effects and Adverse Reactions: There have been no side effects or adverse reactions reported in individuals where proper dosage has been maintained and no complicating illnesses are present.

TAGAMET® (Smith Kline and French Laboratories)

Generic Name: Cimetidine

Dosage Form	Strength	Route
Tablet	200 mg	Oral
	300 mg	
	400 mg	
	800 mg	

When Prescribed: Tagamet is prescribed for the treatment of duodenal ulcers and certain other disorders characterized by an increase in acid secretion in the stomach. It acts by reducing acid secretion in the stomach.

Precautions and Warnings: Tagamet is recommended only for short-term (up to 8 weeks) treatment of ulcers. Nursing mothers should not take this drug.

Side Effects and Adverse Reactions: Diarrhea, muscular pain, dizziness, rash, enlargement of breasts in females, development of breasts in males, confusion.

TALACEN® (Winthrop-Breon Laboratories)

Generic Name: Pentazocine hydrochloride, acetaminophen

Dosage Form	Strength	Route
Tablet	Available in one strength only	Oral

When Prescribed: Talacen is prescribed for relief of mild to moderate pain.

Precautions and Warnings: Patients with a history of drug misuse should not use Talacen because one of the ingredients (pentazocine) has abuse potential. It should not be withdrawn abruptly. Safe use of Talacen in pregnancy has not been established. Caution should be exercised when Talacen is administered to a nursing mother. Safety and effectiveness for children under 12 years have not been established. Talacen may cause sedation, dizziness, or euphoria, so patient should not operate any machinery or drive when using this drug.

Side Effects and Adverse Reactions: Nausea, vomiting, constipation, anorexia, diarrhea, dizziness, lightheadedness, hallucinations, sedation, headache, confusion, disorientation, visual blurring, ringing in the ears, anemia, urinary retention.

TALWIN® Nx (Winthrop Laboratories)

Generic Name: Pentazocine hydrochloride

Dosage Form	Strength	Route
Tablet	50 mg	Oral

When Prescribed: Talwin Nx is a potent analgesic prescribed for the relief of moderate pain when less potent drugs are deemed ineffective.

Precautions and Warnings: Patients using this drug should not drive or operate dangerous machinery. Talwin Nx can be habit forming if overused. Chronic prolonged use of this drug can produce adverse withdrawal symptoms. The safe use of this drug in pregnancy has not been established. Talwin should not be taken by children under 12.

Side Effects and Adverse Reactions: Nausea, vomiting, constipation, abdominal distress, loss of appetite, diarrhea, dizziness, lightheadedness, sedation, euphoria, headache, weakness, disturbed dreams, insomnia, fainting, blurred vision, difficulty focusing, hallucinations, tremor, irritability, excitement, ringing in the ears, sweating, flushing, chills, rash, hives, puffiness of face, decrease in blood pressure, rapid heartbeat, difficulty urinating.

TAVIST® (Sandoz Pharmaceuticals)

Generic Name: Clemastine fumarate

Dosage Form	Strength	Route
Tablet	1.34 mg	Oral
	2.68 mg	Oral
Syrup	0.67 mg/5 ml	Oral

When Prescribed: Tavist is prescribed for relief of symptoms associated with allergic inflammation of nasal mucosa. Tavist tablet 2.68 mg can be prescribed for the treatment of allergic skin conditions.

Precautions and Warnings: All antihistamines and Tavist should be used with caution by patients suffering from glaucoma, asthma, peptic ulcer, thyroid disease, high blood pressure, or urinary bladder neck obstruction. Safety and efficacy of Tavist have not been established for children under 12. Tavist should not be used with other depressants or sleeping pills. Tavist may impair mental alertness, so do not operate any machinery or drive a car when using this drug.

Side Effects and Adverse Reactions: Rash; headache; increase in heart rate; excessive perspiration; chills; dryness of mouth, nose, and throat; sedation; sleepiness; dizziness; disturbed coordination; sleeping disturbances; irritability; convulsions; double vision; loss of appetite; nausea; vomiting; diarrhea; constipation; tightness of chest and wheezing.

TAVIST-D® (Sandoz Pharmaceuticals)

Generic Name: Clemastine fumarate, phenylpropanolamine hydrochloride

Dosage Form	Strength	Route
Tablet	Available in one strength only	Oral

When Prescribed: Tavist-D is prescribed for relief of symptoms associated with allergies, such as sneezing; itching of eyes, nose, or throat; and nasal congestion.

Precautions and Warnings: Tavist-D should not be used by premature infants, newborns, nursing mothers or pregnant women. Efficacy and safety of Tavist-D have not been established for children under 12. Do not take alcohol, sedatives, tranquilizers, or sleeping pills concurrently with Tavist-D unless directed by your physician.

Side Effects and Adverse Reactions: Skin rash; anaphylactic shock; excessive perspiration; chills; dryness of mouth, nose, and throat; hypotension; headache; palpitations; anemia; sedation; sleepiness; dizziness; fatigue; confusion; restlessness; excitation; blurred vision; anorexia; nausea; vomiting; diarrhea; constipation; urinary frequency; difficult urination; urinary retention; early menses.

TEGRETOL® (Geigy Pharmaceuticals)

Generic Name: Carbamazepine

Dosage Form	Strength	Route
Tablet	200 mg	Oral

When Prescribed: Tegretol is prescribed to help control epilepsy in patients who do not respond with other drugs. It is usually used only after other drugs have failed. It may also be prescribed to help control pain arising from a condition known as trigeminal neuralgia.

Precautions and Warnings: This drug may produce fetal defects. This should be kept in mind by epileptic women who are of childbearing potential. It is inadvisable for women to nurse while taking this drug. If dizziness or drowsiness occurs, you should not drive or operate dangerous machinery. This drug should not be abruptly discontinued. The use of this drug requires close monitoring by your physician.

Side Effects and Adverse Reactions: Dizziness, drowsiness, unsteadiness, nausea, vomiting, easy bruising, cuts that do not heal, yellowing of skin or eyes, fever, breathing difficulties, pneumonia, urinary difficulties, impotence, disturbances of coordination, confusion, headache, fatigue, blurred vision, hallucinations, double vision, abnormal eye movements, speech disturbances, abnormal involuntary movements, altered sensation or pain from skin, depression, agitation, talkativeness, ringing in the ears, painful sensitivity to sounds, itching, rash, hives, changes in skin color, increased sensitivity to sunlight, loss of hair, excessive perspiration, gastric upset, abdominal pain, diar-

TENEX® (Robins)

Generic Name: Guanfacine Hydrochloride

Dosage Form	Strength	Route
Tablet	1 mg	Oral

When Prescribed: Tenex is prescribed for the management of hypertension.

Precautions and Warnings: Patients with known allergy to guanfacine hydrochloride should not take Tenex. Tenex should be used with caution in patients with severe heart disease, kidney disease, or liver disease. Sedative effects make driving and operating machinery hazardous. Tenex should be used only if needed in pregnant women and should be avoided by nursing mothers. The safety and effectiveness of Tenex in children under 12 has not been demonstrated and is not recommended.

Side Effects and Adverse Reactions: Usually mild and disappearing after continued use of Tenex the following adverse reactions are common: sedation, dry mouth, weakness, dizziness, constipation, impotence.

Tegretol-(Continued)

rhea, constipation, loss of appetite, dryness of mouth, sore throat, fainting, swelling, conjunctivitis, aching joints and muscles, leg cramps, chills.

TENORETIC® (Stuart Pharmaceuticals)

Generic Name: Atenolol, chlorthalidone

Dosage Form	Strength	Route
Tablet	50 mg	Oral
	100 mg	Oral

When Prescribed: Tenoretic is prescribed to help reduce blood pressure in people with high blood pressure. The "fixed-dose" combination drugs like this are not indicated for starting therapy for high blood pressure.

Precautions and Warnings: Tenoretic should not be used by pregnant or nursing women. Safety and effectiveness for children have not been established. Patients with asthma or other lung diseases should be given this drug with caution.

Side Effects and Adverse Reactions: Slow heart rate, lightheadedness, dizziness, loss of balance, fatigue, lethargy, depression, leg pain, dry eyes, rash, sore throat, disorientation, emotional changes.

TENORMIN® (Stuart Pharmaceuticals)

Generic Name: Atenolol

Dosage Form	Strength	Route
Tablet	50 mg	Oral
	100 mg	

When Prescribed: Tenormin is prescribed to help reduce blood pressure in people with high blood pressure (hypertension).

Precautions and Warnings: The safe use of this drug in pregnancy has not been established. Tenormin is not recommended for nursing mothers or for children.

Side Effects and Adverse Reactions: Slow heartbeat, lightheadedness, dizziness, loss of balance, tiredness, fatigue, lethargy, drowsiness, depression, cold extremities, leg pain, vivid dreams, diarrhea, nausea, wheezing, breathing difficulties, rash, dry eyes, bruising, fever, sore throat, visual disturbances, hallucinations, disorientation, memory loss, emotional changes.

TENUATE® DOSPAN® (Merrell-National Laboratories)

Generic Name: Diethylpropion hydrochloride

Dosage Form	Strength	Route
Tablet	25 mg	Oral
Dospan® tablet (Time Release)	75 mg	Oral

When Prescribed: Tenuate Dospan is a prolonged-action tablet containing a drug which is used for weight reduction in overweight individuals who cannot lose sufficient weight by diet alone. It is usually prescribed for a short period of time (a few weeks), during which time diet is controlled.

Precautions and Warnings: Tenuate is a stimulant which may impair judgment. Patients should use caution in driving or operating machinery. Tenuate is related to amphetamines, which have a potential for abuse resulting in physical and/or psychological dependence. Tenuate should not be taken by children under 12.

Side Effects and Adverse Reactions: Irregular heartbeat, high blood pressure, overstimulation, restlessness, dizziness, insomnia, changes in mood, tremor, headache, psychotic episodes, dryness of mouth, unpleasant taste, diarrhea, constipation, gastrointestinal pain, hives, impotence, changes in sex drive, drowsiness, nervousness, anxiety, nausea, vomiting, diarrhea, constipation, rash, development of breasts in males, enlargement of breasts, menstrual difficulties, breathing difficulties, hair loss, muscle pain, urinary difficulties, increased sweating.

TERAZOL 7® (Ortho Pharmaceutical)

Generic Name: Terconazole

Dosage Form	Strength	Route
Cream	.4%	Vaginal

When Prescribed: Terazol 7 is a vaginal cream prescribed to treat monilia (yeast) infections of the vaginal tract.

Precautions and Warnings: Patients known to be allergic to terconazole or any component of the cream should not use Terazol 7. Discontinue use and call your doctor if irritation, fever, chills, or flulike symptoms occur. If there is no response to Terazol 7, test should be repeated to confirm diagnosis. Pregnant and nursing mothers should avoid use of Terazol 7.

Side Effects and Adverse Reactions: Headaches and body pain, burning, itching, irritation.

TERPIN HYDRATE WITH CO-DEINE
The generic name for a drug produced by numerous companies.

Dosage Form	Strength	Route
Elixir	Available in one strength only	Oral

When Prescribed: Elixir Terpin Hydrate with Codeine is prescribed for coughs accompanying colds and allergies.

Precautions and Warnings: Elixir Terpin Hydrate with Codeine causes drowsiness in some people. Patients who become drowsy should not drive or engage in activities requiring alert responses. Sleeping pills, sedatives, alcohol, or tranquilizers should not be used with this drug. This drug contains codeine, which may be habit forming.

Side Effects and Adverse Reactions: Dry mouth, blurred vision, thirst, dizziness, drowsiness, confusion, nervousness, restlessness, nausea, vomiting, diarrhea, constipation, tingling, nasal stuffiness, headache, insomnia, low blood pressure, heartburn.

TESSALON® (DuPont Pharmaceuticals, Inc.)

Generic Name: Benzonatate

Dosage Form	Strength	Route
Perles	100 mg	Oral

When Prescribed: Tessalon is prescribed for relief of coughing.

Precautions and Warnings: The safe use of this drug by pregnant and nursing women has not been established. Tessalon perles (fluid-filled capsules) should not be chewed or crushed.

Side Effects and Adverse Reactions: Sedation, headache, mild dizziness, nasal congestion, constipation, gastrointestinal upset, burning in eyes, numbness in chest.

TETRACYCLINE

The generic name for a drug produced by numerous companies in various forms and strengths. Also marketed as:
ACHROMYCIN® Lederle;
KESSO-TETRA® McKesson;
ROBITET® SYRUP Robins;
SK-TETRACYCLINE® SYRUP Smith Kline and French;
SUMYCIN® SYRUP Squibb.

Generic Name: Tetracycline hydrochloride

Dosage Form	Strength	Route
Capsule	250 mg	Oral
	500 mg	Oral
Tablet	250 mg	Oral
	500 mg	Oral
Syrup	125 mg/5 cc	Oral

When Prescribed: Tetracycline is an effective antibiotic prescribed for many different types of infection. It is often used in place of penicillin in patients who are allergic to penicillin.

Precautions and Warnings: Tetracycline should not be taken by people overly sensitive to this drug. If any of the side effects listed below occur, consult your physician immediately. Not recommended for pregnant women, infants, or children under the age of 8.

Side Effects and Adverse Reactions: Exaggerated sunburn, superinfection by nonsusceptible organisms, loss of appetite, nausea, vomiting, diarrhea, inflammation of the tongue, difficulty swallowing, stomach pains, inflammation of the bowel and genital region, skin rash, hives, swelling, fainting.

THEO-DUR® (Key Pharmaceuticals, Inc.)

Generic Name: Theophylline (anhydrous)

Dosage Form	Strength	Route
Sustained release Tablet	100 mg 200 mg 300 mg	Oral

When Prescribed: Theo-Dur is prescribed for the relief and/or prevention of asthma and breathing difficulties associated with chronic bronchitis or emphysema.

Precautions and Warnings: Theo-Dur tablets should not be chewed or crushed so they can dissolve slowly into the system. The safe use of this drug in pregnancy has not been established.

Side Effects and Adverse Reactions: Nausea, vomiting, heartburn, blood in vomit, diarrhea, headache, irritability, restlessness, insomnia, heightened reflexes, muscle twitches, convulsions, heart flutters, rapid heartbeat, flushing of skin, low blood pressure, rapid breathing, increased urination.

THEO-DUR SPRINKLE® (Key Pharmaceuticals, Inc.)

Generic Name: Theophylline (anhydrous)

Dosage Form	Strength	Route
Capsule	50 mg	Oral
	75 mg	Oral
	125 mg	Oral
	200 mg	Oral

When Prescribed: Theo-Dur Sprinkle capsules are prescribed for the relief and/or prevention of asthma and breathing difficulties associated with chronic bronchitis or emphysema.

Precautions and Warnings: Theo-Dur Sprinkle capsules dissolve slowly into the system. The safe use of this drug in pregnancy has not been established.

Side Effects and Adverse Reactions: Nausea, vomiting, heartburn, blood in vomit, diarrhea, headache, irritability, restlessness, insomnia, heightened reflexes, muscle twitches, convulsions, heart flutters, rapid heartbeat, flushing of skin, low blood pressure, rapid breathing, increased urination.

THORAZINE® (Smith Kline and French Laboratories)

Generic Name: Chlorpromazine

Dosage Form	Strength	Route
Tablet	10 mg	Oral
	25 mg	Oral
	50 mg	Oral
	100 mg	Oral
	200 mg	Oral
Capsule (Time	30 mg	Oral
Release)	75 mg	Oral
(Spansules®)	150 mg	Oral
	200 mg	Oral
	300 mg	Oral
Liquid	10 mg/5 ml	Oral
Suppository	25 mg	Rectal
	100 mg	Rectal

When Prescribed: Thorazine is a sedative prescribed for the management of certain types of mental illness, for the control of nausea and vomiting, for chronic hiccups, to control overactive children and in other instances where a reduction of anxiety or apprehension is desirable.

Precautions and Warnings: This drug may impair mental and/or physical abilities. Patients taking Thorazine should not drive or operate machinery. This drug should not be used with alcohol, tranquilizers, sleeping pills or sedatives. The safe use of this drug in pregnancy has not been established.

Side Effects and Adverse Reactions: Drowsiness, yellow skin or eyes, anemia, sore throat, low blood pressure, fainting, tremors, abnormal movements, abnormal facial movements or expression, skin eruptions, hives, breast enlargement, lactation, false positive pregnancy tests, lack of menstruation, breast growth in males, dry mouth, nasal con-

THYROID TABLETS
The generic name for a drug produced by numerous companies in various strengths.

Generic Name: Thyroid hormone

Dosage Form	Strength	Route
Tablet	15 mg	Oral
	30 mg	Oral
	60 mg	Oral
	90 mg	Oral
	120 mg	Oral

When Prescribed: Thyroid tablets supply thyroid hormone either from natural or synthetic sources. Thyroid tablets are prescribed when the body produces insufficient thyroid hormone. This can be due to a variety of reasons, some of which are surgery, disease, birth defect, and radiation.

Precautions and Warnings: Thyroid therapy should be closely regulated by your physician.

Side Effects and Adverse Reactions: There have been no side effects or adverse reactions reported in individuals when proper dosage has been maintained and no complicating illnesses are present. Overdosage can result in irregular heartbeat, increased heart rate, weight loss, chest pains, tremors, headache, diarrhea, nervousness, insomnia, sweating, intolerance to heat and fever.

TIGAN® (Beecham Laboratories)

Generic Name: Trimethobenzamide hydrochloride

Dosage Form	Strength	Route
Suppository (Pediatric)	100 mg	Rectal
Suppository	200 mg	Rectal
Capsule	100 mg	Oral
	250 mg	Oral

When Prescribed: Tigan is prescribed for the control of nausea and vomiting. The suppository is particularly effective for frequent or prolonged vomiting when the oral dose may be regurgitated.

Precautions and Warnings: Since drowsiness may occur, patients should not drive or operate machinery. The safe use of Tigan in pregnancy has not been established.

Side Effects and Adverse Reactions: Tremors, jerky movements, blurring of vision, coma, convulsion, depression of mood, diarrhea, disorientation, dizziness, drowsiness, headache, yellow skin or eyes, muscle cramps, allergic skin reactions.

Thorazine-(Continued)

gestion, constipation, inability to urinate, dilation of pupils, jaundice, changes in eyes, fever.

TIMOPTIC® (Merck Sharp and Dohme)

Generic Name: Timolol maleate

Dosage Form	Strength	Route
Solution (Eye Drop)	0.25%	Eye Drop
	0.50%	Eye Drop

When Prescribed: Timoptic is prescribed to lower elevated pressure in the eye that results from various disorders including glaucoma.

Precautions and Warnings: This drug is not recommended for use in children.

Side Effects and Adverse Reactions: Eye irritation, rash, reduction of heart rate.

TOBREX® (Alcon Inc.)

Generic Name: Tobramycin

Dosage Form	Strength	Route
Liquid	0.3%	Intraocular (eye drop)
Ointment	0.3%	Intraocular (eye ointment)

When Prescribed: Tobrex is prescribed for treatment of eye infections.

Precautions and Warnings: Prolonged use of Tobrex should be avoided, as with other antibiotics, to prevent overgrowth of nonsusceptible organisms. It should be avoided by pregnant women and nursing mothers.

Side Effects and Adverse Reactions: Eyelid itching, swelling, redness.

TOFRANIL® (Geigy Pharmaceuticals)

Generic Name: Imipramine hydrochloride

Dosage Form	Strength	Route
Tablet	10 mg	Oral
	25 mg	Oral
	50 mg	Oral

When Prescribed: Tofranil is prescribed for the relief of symptoms of depression. It may also be prescribed to control daytime frequency of urination and to control bed-wetting in individuals older than 6.

Precautions and Warnings: This drug can impair mental and/or physical abilities. Alcohol should not be used with this drug. Tofranil can lead to serious and sometimes fatal reactions if taken with certain other drugs. Be sure to inform your physician of all drugs you take. Mothers should not nurse while taking this drug.

Side Effects and Adverse Reactions: Changes in blood pressure, irregular heartbeat, stroke, fainting, confusion, hallucinations, disorientation, delusions, anxiety, restlessness, agitation, insomnia, nightmares, numbness or tingling sensation, incoordination, loss of balance, tremors, ringing in the ears, dry mouth, blurred vision, trouble adapting to changing light, dilation of pupils, constipation, difficulty urinating, allergic skin disorders, anemia, sore throat, nausea, vomiting, heartburn, strange taste, abdominal cramps, black tongue, breast enlargement in males, breast enlargement and lactation in females, change in sexual behavior, swelling of testicles, yellow skin or eyes, change in weight, perspiration, frequent urination, dizziness, weakness, fatigue, loss of appetite, diarrhea, black tongue, loss of hair.

TOLECTIN® (McNeil Laboratories, Inc.)

Generic Name: Tolmetin Sodium

Dosage Form	Strength	Route
Capsule	400 mg	Oral
Tablet	200 mg	Oral

When Prescribed: Tolectin is prescribed for the relief of pain and inflammation of arthritis. It is as effective as aspirin in reducing pain and inflammation but is usually better tolerated in the stomach.

Precautions and Warnings: This drug is not recommended for pregnant women or nursing mothers.

Side Effects and Adverse Reactions: Nausea, indigestion, abdominal pain, gastrointestinal distress, gas, diarrhea, constipation, vomiting, stomach upset, headache, weakness, chest pain, fainting, swelling, dizziness, lightheadedness, nervousness, drowsiness, insomnia, depression, skin rash, itching, skin irritation, ringing in the ears.

TOLINASE® (The Upjohn Company)

Generic Name: Tolazamide

Dosage Form	Strength	Route
Tablet	100 mg	Oral
	250 mg	Oral
	500 mg	Oral

When Prescribed: Tolinase is prescribed for diabetes (diabetes mellitus) to control the blood sugar levels in addition to diet. It is prescribed after a sufficient trial of dietary therapy has proved unsatisfactory. Tolinase can replace the need for insulin by helping to release the body's own insulin.

Precautions and Warnings: Blood and urine glucose should be monitored periodically while using Tolinase. The effect of decreasing blood-sugar levels can be potentiated by other drugs. Inform your physician before starting any other medication. Drinking alcohol can result in severe vomiting and abdominal cramps. Tolinase should be used during pregnancy only if the potential benefit justifies the potential risk to the fetus and should be discontinued at least one month prior to the expected delivery date. Safety and effectiveness for children's use of this drug has not been established. Tolinase does not replace the need to restrict diet.

Side Effects and Adverse Reactions: Jaundice, nausea, heartburn, skin rashes, different types of anemia, hypoglycemia (low blood sugar levels), diarrhea, constipation, abdominal pain, gas, itching, weakness, fatigue, loss of balance, drowsiness, dizziness, depression, headache.

TOPICORT® (Hoechst-Roussel Pharmaceuticals, Inc.)

Generic Name: Desoximetasone

Dosage Form	Strength	Route
Emollient Cream	0.25%	Topical (apply directly to affected area)
Emollient Cream	0.05%	Same as above
Gel	0.05%	Same as above
Ointment	0.25%	Same as above

When Prescribed: Topicort is prescribed for relief of inflammatory and itching conditions which respond to corticosteroids.

Precautions and Warnings: Topicort is to be used as directed by the physician. It is for external use only. Avoid contact with eyes. The treated skin area should not be bandaged or otherwise covered or wrapped so as to be occlusive unless directed by the physician. Parents of pediatric patients should not use tight diapers or plastic pants on a child being treated in the diaper area, as these garments may constitute occlusive dressings. Topicort is a corticosteroid, and this group of drugs is not prescribed for pregnant or nursing women.

Side Effects and Adverse Reactions: Burning, itching, irritation, dryness, inflammation of hair follicles, secondary infection, shrinkage of skin.

TRANSDERM-NITRO® (Ciba Pharmaceutical Company)

Generic Name: Nitroglycerin

Dosage Form	Strength	Route
Patch	2.5 mg	Local
	5 mg	Local
	10 mg	Local
	15 mg	Local

When Prescribed: Transderm-Nitro is prescribed for prevention and treatment of angina pectoris (chest pains due to decreased blood flow to the heart).

Precautions and Warnings: Transderm-Nitro should not be withdrawn immediately. Instructions about using the patch and other necessary information are given in a leaflet with the medication.

Side Effects and Adverse Reactions: Hypotension, headache, increase in heart rate, flushing, dizziness, nausea, vomiting, inflammation of the skin.

TRANSDERM-SCOP® (Formerly TRANSDERM-V) (Ciba Pharmaceutical Company)

Generic Name: Scopolamine

Dosage Form	Strength	Route
Disc	Available in one strength only	Apply to skin in back of ear

When Prescribed: Transderm-Scop is prescribed for prevention of nausea and vomiting associated with motion sickness in adults.

Precautions and Warnings: The disc should be applied only to skin in back of the ear. Transderm-Scop should not be used by patients with glaucoma. It should not be used by children and should be used with caution by the elderly. There are possibilities of becoming disoriented, drowsy, and confused after using this product, so do not engage in activities which require mental alertness. Do not operate dangerous machinery. Pregnant and nursing women should use it with great caution.

Side Effects and Adverse Reactions: Dryness of mouth; drowsiness; visual problems such as blurred vision, dilation of pupils; disorientation; memory disturbances; dizziness; restlessness; hallucinations; confusion; difficult urination; itchy or red eyes.

TRANXENE® (Abbott Laboratories)

Generic Name: Clorazepate dipotassium

Dosage Form	Strength	Route
Capsule	3.75 mg	Oral
	7.5 mg	Oral
Capsule	22.5	Oral
(Time Release)	15.0 mg	Oral
	11.25	Oral
Tablet	3.75 mg	Oral
	7.5 mg	Oral
	15.0 mg	Oral

When Prescribed: Tranxene is prescribed for the relief of anxiety resulting from neurotic conditions as well as anxiety which can accompany diseases.

Precautions and Warnings: Patients taking this drug should not drive or operate machinery. Tranxene should not be taken with alcohol, sedatives, tranquilizers or sleeping pills. A physical and/or psychological dependence on Tranxene can occur. This drug is not recommended for pregnant women or nursing mothers.

Side Effects and Adverse Reactions: Drowsiness, dizziness, gastrointestinal complaints, nervousness, blurred vision, dry mouth, headache, mental confusion, insomnia, rash, fatigue, loss of balance, urinary difficulties, irritability, double vision, depression, slurred speech.

TRENTAL® (Hoechst-Roussel Pharmaceuticals, Inc.)

Generic Name: Pentoxifylline

Dosage Form	Strength	Route
Tablet	400 mg	Oral

When Prescribed: Trental is a drug which can increase blood flow to certain areas of the body. It is prescribed for patients suffering from intermittent muscle pain due to arterial disease.

Precautions and Warnings: Trental can improve function and symptoms but is not intended to replace more definitive therapy, such as surgical bypass or other appropriate surgical procedures. It should be avoided by pregnant and nursing women. Safety and effectiveness for children under 18 have not been established.

Side Effects and Adverse Reactions: The incidence of adverse reactions was higher in the capsule studies than in the tablet studies. Side effects are flushing, dyspepsia, nausea, dizziness, headache, and blurred vision.

TRIAMCINOLONE ACETONIDE The

generic name for a drug produced by numerous companies in various forms and strengths.

Dosage Form	Strength	Route
Cream	0.025%	Topical
	0.1%	(apply
	0.5%	directly to
		affected
		area)
Ointment	0.1%	Topical
	0.5%	(apply
		directly to
		the affected
		area)

When Prescribed: Triamcinolone acetonide is a local steroid which reduces inflammation, itching, and swelling associated with skin disorders.

Precautions and Warnings: Triamcinolone acetonide should not be used in the eyes. The treated area should not be bandaged or wrapped by occlusive dressings. This drug should not be used in large amounts by pregnant patients or for prolonged periods of time. Prolonged use of this drug by children may interfere with their growth and development.

Side Effects and Adverse Reactions: Burning, itching, irritation, infected hair follicles, dryness, increased hair growth, acne, loss of pigmentation, skin damage.

TRIAVIL® (Merck Sharp and Dohme)

Generic Name: Perphenazine, amitriptyline hydrochloride

Dosage Form	Strength	Route
Tablet	2–25	Oral
	4–25	Oral
	2–10	Oral
	4–10	Oral

When Prescribed: Triavil is prescribed for various psychological problems characterized by anxiety and depression. This drug is used to control a wide variety of mental disorders.

Precautions and Warnings: Patients using this drug should not drive or operate machinery. Triavil should not be taken with alcohol, sedatives, sleeping pills or tranquilizers. This drug is not recommended for use in pregnant patients, nursing mothers, or in children.

Side Effects and Adverse Reactions: Tremors, jerky movements, skin eruptions, hives, rash, increased sensitivity to sunlight, asthma, fainting, swelling, lactation, breast enlargement (male and female), menstrual disturbances, excitement, changes in blood pressure, rapid heartbeat, dry mouth, salivation, headache, loss of appetite, nausea, vomiting, constipation, urinary frequency, blurred vision, nasal congestion, increased appetite, convulsions, change of skin color, impotence, yellow skin or eyes, eye disorders, nightmares, numbness or tingling, insomnia, loss of balance, ringing in ears, fatigue, dizziness, drowsiness, abnormal, uncontrollable movements of tongue or face, black tongue, loss of appetite, increased perspiration, loss of hair.

TRIDESILON® (Miles Pharmaceuticals)

Generic Name: Desonide

Dosage Form	Strength	Route
Cream	0.05%	Topical (apply directly to affected area)
Ointment	0.05%	Topical

When Prescribed: Tridesilone is a topical corticosteroid which reduces inflammation, itching, and swelling associated with skin disorders.

Precautions and Warnings: Avoid contact with eyes. The treated skin area should not be bandaged or otherwise covered or wrapped. Patients should report to their physician any sign of local skin abnormality. Parents of pediatric patients should be advised not to use tight-fitting diapers or plastic pants on a child treated in the diaper area. Tridesilon should not be used extensively by pregnant patients in large amounts or for prolonged periods of time.

Side Effects and Adverse Reactions: Burning, itching, irritation, dryness, decrease in pigmentation.

TRILAFON® (Schering Corporation)

Generic Name: Perphenazine

Dosage Form	Strength	Route
Tablet	4 mg	Oral
	8 mg	Oral
	16 mg	Oral
Liquid	16 mg/5 ml	Oral

When Prescribed: Trilafon is prescribed for management of manifestations of emotional problems and for control of severe nausea and vomiting in adults.

Precautions and Warnings: Rise in body temperature suggests intolerance to Trilafon. In this case, it should be discontinued. High doses of Trilafon may decrease blood pressure. It is suggested to avoid alcohol and other depressants (antihistamines, barbiturates) while taking Trilafon.

Side Effects and Adverse Reactions: Tardive dyskinesia (a condition in which patient shows involuntary muscular movements), aches, numbness of certain parts of the body, discoloration of the tongue, tight feeling in throat, slurred speech.

TRI-LEVLEN 28® (Berlex)

Generic Name: Levonorgestrel and Ethinyl Estradiol

Dosage Form	Strength	Route
Tablet	Available in one strength only	Oral

When Prescribed: Tri-Levlen 28 is an oral contraceptive prescribed for the prevention of pregnancy.

Precautions and Warnings: Contraceptives should not be used by women susceptible to blood clotting, cerebrolvascular or coronary artery disease, suspected cancer of the breast, tumors, undiagnosed genital bleeding, known or suspected pregnancy, or liver tumor developed during use of estrogen. Women using oral contraceptives should not smoke. Cigarette smoking increases the risk for serious cardiovascular side effects. Use of oral contraceptives increases the risk of several serious conditions: blood clot, stroke, heart attack, liver disease, gallbladder disease, hypertension. A completed medical and family history should be taken and evaluated prior to the initiation of oral contraception. Regular physical examinations and pap smears should be taken. Nursing mothers should take oral contraceptives with caution. A booklet has been provided for your information. Ask your physician for this booklet.

Side Effects and Adverse Reactions: Birth defects, nausea, vomiting, breakthrough bleeding, spotting, change in menstrual flow, painful or suppressed

TRIMETHOPRIM WITH SULFAMETHOXAZOLE
The generic name for a drug produced by numerous companies in various forms and strengths. Also marketed as:
BACTRIM® Roche;
SEPTRA® Burroughs Wellcome;
COTRIM® Lemon.

Dosage Form	Strength	Route
Tablet	Regular strength	Oral
Tablet	Double strength	Oral
Suspension	Available in one strength only	Oral

When Prescribed: Trimethoprim with sulfamethoxazole is a combination of drugs prescribed for the treatment of certain types of urinary tract infections and for certain other types of bacterial infections.

Precautions and Warnings: Trimethoprim with sulfamethoxazole is not recommended during pregnancy or for nursing mothers. If any of the side effects or adverse reactions listed below appear, consult your physician.

Side Effects and Adverse Reactions: Rash, sore throat, stomach upset, nausea, vomiting, abdominal pains, diarrhea, yellowing of skin, headache, body aches, depression, dizziness, fever, chills, urinary difficulties.

Tri-levlen 28-(Continued)

menstruation, temporary infertility, tender, enlarged, and secreting breast, changes in weight, change in cervical erosion and cervical secretion, rash, mental depression.

TRIMOX® (Squib)

Generic Name: Amoxicillin

Dosage Form	Strength	Route
Capsule	250 mg	Oral
	500 mg	Oral
Suspension	125 mg	Oral
	250 mg	Oral

When Prescribed: Trimox is used in the treatment of numerous susceptible bacterial infections including infections of the ear, nose, and throat, and gonorrhea.

Precautions and Warnings: Serious allergic reactions are more likely to occur in susceptible individuals. Inform your physician of any previous allergic reactions to antibiotics; discontinue use and call your physician immediately if any side effects occur. Diabetic patients should notify physician of any plan to change diet or dosage of diabetic medication.

Side Effects and Adverse Reactions: Black "hairy" tongue, nausea, vomiting, diarrhea, skin rash, anemia, sore mouth, superinfection.

TRINALIN™ REPETABS® (Schering Corporation)

Generic Name: Azatadine maleate, pseudoephedrine sulfate

Dosage Form	Strength	Route
Tablet	Available in one strength only	Oral

When Prescribed: Trinalin Repetabs is prescribed for relief of symptoms of upper respiratory congestion, allergic rhinitis, and nasal congestion.

Precautions and Warnings: Trinalin Repetabs should be used with caution by patients with peptic ulcers, urinary bladder obstruction, cardiovascular disease, and diabetes, and patients using digoxin. Trinalin Repetabs may cause drowsiness, and patients should not engage in activities requiring mental alertness, such as driving or operating machinery. This medication should not be given to children under 12.

Side Effects and Adverse Reactions: Drowsiness; skin rash; anaphylactic shock; excessive perspiration; chills; dryness of mouth, throat, and nose; hypertension; hypotension; headache; palpitations; anemia; sedation; sleepiness; dizziness; confusion; restlessness; insomnia; blurred vision; convulsions; anxiety; depression.

TRIPHASIL 28® (Wyeth Laboratories)

Generic Name: Levonorgestrel, ethinyl estradiol

Dosage Form	Strength	Route
Tablet	Available in one strength only	Oral

When Prescribed: Triphasil is a comparatively new oral contraceptive. It is prescribed for birth control. It contains different color tablets for different phases of the menstrual cycle.

Precautions and Warnings: Whenever you start any of the contraceptives (oral), read patient information leaflet carefully. Oral contraceptives are powerful and effective drugs which can have serious side effects, including: blood clots, unusual bleeding, stroke, heart attack, liver tumors, gallbladder disease, and high blood pressure. Safe use of this drug requires a discussion with your physician. Cigarette smoking increases the risk of cardiovascular side effects. If any of the following symptoms occur, consult your physician immediately.

Side Effects and Adverse Reactions: Nausea; vomiting; abdominal cramps; bloating; bleeding or spotting at times other than during menstruation; change in menstrual flow; pain associated with menstruation; absence of menstruation; temporary infertility after discontinuing treatment; swelling; abnormal darkening of the skin; breast changes including tenderness, enlargement, and secretion; increase or decrease in body weight; change in vaginal secretions; reduction in amount of breast milk if taken after childbirth; yellowing of skin or eyes; headaches; rash; depression; vaginal infections; cramps; difficulty with contact

TRI-VI-FLOR® (Mead Johnson Nutritional Division)

Generic Name: Vitamins A, D, C, Fluoride

Dosage Form	Strength	Route
Liquid	0.25 mg	Oral
	0.5 mg	Oral
Tablet	1 mg	Oral
	0.5 mg	Oral

When Prescribed: Tri-Vi-Flor is prescribed for infants and children to prevent vitamin deficiencies and to supply fluoride for the prevention of tooth decay in areas where the fluoride content of the water is low.

Precautions and Warnings: Tri-Vi-Flor should only be used in areas where the fluoride content of the drinking water is below 0.7 parts per million. Do not give more than prescribed. Keep out of reach of children.

Side Effects and Adverse Reactions: Overuse can lead to fluoride poisoning. Rash may develop in children allergic to this preparation.

Triphasil 28-(Continued)

lenses; visual difficulties; uncontrollable body movements; change in sex drive; change in appetite; nervousness; dizziness; increase of facial hair; loss of scalp hair; itching; skin eruptions.

TUSSEND® (Merrell Dow Pharmaceuticals, Inc.)

Generic Name: Hydrocodone bitartrate, pseudoephedrine hydrochloride, alcohol (liquid only)

Dosage Form	Strength	Route
Liquid	Both forms available in one strength only	Oral
Tablet		Oral

When Prescribed: Tussend is prescribed for the control of cough resulting from respiratory infections.

Precautions and Warnings: Tussend contains a narcotic that may be habit forming. Prolonged or excessive use can result in physical and/or psychological dependence. Do not take with alcohol, tranquilizers, sedatives or sleeping pills unless directed by your physician. If drowsiness occurs, you should not drive or operate dangerous machinery. The safe use of this drug in pregnant females has not been established. Tussend should not be taken by nursing mothers.

Side Effects and Adverse Reactions: Gastrointestinal upset, nausea, drowsiness, constipation, heart flutters, rapid heartbeat, headache, dizziness, fear, anxiety, tenseness, restlessness, tremor, weakness, pallor, respiratory problems, urinary problems, insomnia, hallucinations, convulsions.

TUSSIONEX® (Pennwalt)

Generic Name: Resin complexes of hydrocodone and phenyltoloxamine

Dosage Form	Strength	Route
Capsule	All forms available in one strength only	Oral
Tablet		Oral
Liquid		Oral

When Prescribed: Tussionex is prescribed for the control of coughing.

Precautions and Warnings: Do not exceed recommended dosage. If cough continues despite the recommended dosage, contact your physician. Not to be taken with alcohol.

Side Effects and Adverse Reactions: Constipation, nausea, facial itching, drowsiness.

TUSSI-ORGANIDIN® (Wallace Laboratories)

Generic Name: Iodinated glycerol, codeine phosphate

Dosage Form	Strength	Route
Liquid	Available in one strength only	Oral

When Prescribed: Tussi-Organidin is prescribed for the control of cough resulting from a variety of disorders.

Precautions and Warnings: This compound contains codeine, which may be habit-forming. If drowsiness occurs, you should not drive or operate dangerous machinery. This drug should not be taken with alcohol, tranquilizers, sleeping pills, sedatives, or other nervous system depressants unless directed by your physician. This drug should not be taken by pregnant women or nursing mothers.

Side Effects and Adverse Reactions: Abdominal pain, rash, enlarged thyroid, painful salivary glands, nausea, vomiting, constipation, drowsiness, dizziness, dry mouth, headache, heartburn, urinary disturbances, visual disturbances, excitation.

TUSSI-ORGANIDIN DM® (Wallace Laboratories)

Generic Name: Organidine, dextromethorphan hydrobromide

Dosage Form	Strength	Route
Liquid	Available in one strength only	Oral

When Prescribed: Tussi-Organidin DM is prescribed for symptomatic relief of irritating, nonproductive cough associated with respiratory tract conditions such as chronic bronchitis, asthma, and the common cold.

Precautions and Warnings: Tussi-Organidin DM should not be used by patients who have a history of sensitivity to iodides, pregnant women, nursing mothers, or newborns.

Side Effects and Adverse Reactions: Gastrointestinal irritation; hypersensitivity; drowsiness; dry mouth, throat, and nose.

TUSS-ORNADE® (Smith Kline and French Laboratories)

Generic Name: Caramiphen edisylate, phenylpropanolamine hydrochloride

Dosage Form	Strength	Route
Capsule (Spansules®)	Available in one strength only	Oral
Liquid (contains alcohol)	Available in one strength only	Oral

When Prescribed: Tuss-Ornade is prescribed for relief from coughing, upper respiratory congestion, and "runny nose" associated with the common cold, sinus infections and allergies.

Precautions and Warnings: Tuss-Ornade should not be taken with certain drugs prescribed for high blood pressure. If drowsiness or blurred vision occurs, you should not operate a car or machinery or participate in activities where alertness is required.

Side Effects and Adverse Reactions: Nausea, vomiting, dry mouth, nervousness, dizziness, headache, drowsiness, visual disturbances, mental confusion, painful urination, skin disorders, diarrhea, rash, chest pain, heart flutters, tremors, convulsions, dryness of nose, insomnia, abdominal pain, loss of coordination, loss of appetite, constipation.

TYLENOL® with CODEINE (McNeil Laboratories, Inc.)

Generic Name: Acetaminophen, codeine

Dosage Form	Strength	Route
Tablet	No. 1	Oral
	No. 2	Oral
	No. 3	Oral
	No. 4	Oral
Elixir (contains alcohol)	Available in one strength only	Oral
Capsule	No. 1	Oral
	No. 2	Oral
	No. 3	Oral
	No. 4	Oral

When Prescribed: Tylenol with codeine is prescribed for the relief of pain of various causes, and for the relief of aches, pain and coughing that may be symptoms of colds or flu.

Precautions and Warnings: Tylenol with codeine contains a narcotic pain reliever which may be habit forming. This preparation may cause drowsiness. Therefore driving motor vehicles or operating dangerous machinery is discouraged while taking this treatment.

Side Effects and Adverse Reactions: Drowsiness, constipation, nausea, lightheadedness, dizziness, vomiting, mood changes, itching, rash.

TYLOX® (McNeil Pharmaceutical)

Generic Name: Oxycodone hydrochloride, oxycodone terephthalate, acetaminophen

Dosage Form	Strength	Route
Capsule	Available in one strength only	Oral

When Prescribed: Tylox is prescribed for the relief of moderate to moderately severe pain.

Precautions and Warnings: This drug can possibly be physically addictive. Psychological dependence and tolerance (a larger dose is necessary to produce the same effect) can also occur. Patients taking this drug may become drowsy. If so, you should not drive or operate dangerous machinery. Tylox should not be taken with alcohol, tranquilizers, sleeping pills or sedatives unless specifically directed by your physician. The safe use of this drug in pregnant women, nursing mothers and children has not been established.

Side Effects and Adverse Reactions: Lightheadedness, dizziness, sedation, nausea, vomiting, mood changes, constipation, itching, skin rash.

ULTRACEF® (Bristol Laboratories)

Generic Name: Cefadroxil

Dosage Form	Strength	Route
Tablet	1 gm	Oral
Capsule	500 mg	Oral
Capsule	1 gm	Oral
Suspension	125 mg/5 ml	Oral
Suspension	250 mg/5 ml	Oral

When Prescribed: Ultracef is an antibiotic prescribed for a variety of infections including those of the skin and urogenital and respiratory tracts.

Precautions and Warnings: People who are allergic to penicillin are often allergic to Ultracef. Consult your physician if any side effects or adverse reactions occur. It should be used with caution by pregnant women and nursing mothers.

Side Effects and Adverse Reactions: Nausea (administration with food will decrease nausea), vomiting, diarrhea, inflammation of urogenital area.

URISED® (Webcon Pharmaceuticals)

Generic Name: Methanamine, phenyl salicylate, methylene blue, benzoic acid, atropine sulfate, hyoscyamine

Dosage Form	Strength	Route
Tablet	Available in one strength only	Oral

When Prescribed: Urised is prescribed for relief of discomfort of the lower urinary tract caused by increased movement resulting from inflammation or diagnostic procedures. It can be used for inflammation of the bladder, urethra, and some other parts of the urinary tract.

Precautions and Warnings: Do not exceed recommended dose. Do not use with any other drug which belongs to a sulfa group. Drugs and foods which increase urinary pH should not be used. The urine may become blue to blue-green and the feces may be discolored as a result of excretion of methylene blue. In pregnancy, Urised should be used only if it is clearly needed. Caution should be exercised by nursing mothers. In children under 12, the dose should be adjusted according to the age and weight of the patient.

Side Effects and Adverse Reactions: If severe dryness of mouth, flushing, or difficulty in initiating urination occurs, decrease the dose. If pulse rate increases or dizziness or blurring of vision occurs, discontinue the drug immediately.

VALISONE® (Schering Corporation)

Generic Name: Betamethasone valerate

Dosage Form	Strength	Route
Cream	.01% .1%	Topical (all forms are applied directly to affected area)
Ointment	.1%	
Lotion	.1%	

When Prescribed: Valisone is a potent steroidal drug which is prescribed for the relief of pain, itching and inflammation caused by conditions such as allergic reactions.

Precautions and Warnings: Not for use in the eyes. Valisone should not be used extensively or for prolonged periods in pregnant women.

Side Effects and Adverse Reactions: Burning, itching, irritation, dryness, hair follicle infection, hair growth, pimples, loss of skin color, skin decay, infection.

VALIUM® (Roche Laboratories)

Generic Name: Diazepam

Dosage Form	Strength	Route
Tablet	2 mg	Oral
	5 mg	Oral
	10 mg	Oral

When Prescribed: Valium is prescribed for a wide variety of problems to provide relief from tension and anxiety. It is used in a wide variety of physical and/or psychological disorders. It is often prescribed along with other drugs for the relief of muscle or skeletal disorders or for the prevention of convulsions. It is helpful in preventing reactions during withdrawal in alcoholics.

Precautions and Warnings: Patients taking this drug should not drive or operate machinery. Valium should not be taken with alcohol, sedatives, tranquilizers or sleeping pills. A physical and/or psychological dependence on Valium can occur. The use of Valium during pregnancy should almost always be avoided.

Side Effects and Adverse Reactions: Drowsiness, fatigue, loss of balance, confusion, constipation, depression, double vision, aches in joints, fainting, frequent urination, yellowing of skin or eyes, changes in sex drive, nausea, changes in salivation, skin rash, slurred speech, tremors, lack of urination, dizziness, blurred vision, anxiety, hallucinations, muscle spasticity, insomnia, rage, sleep disturbances.

VANCENASE® (Schering Corporation)

Generic Name: Beclomethasone dipropionate

Dosage Form	Strength	Route
Inhaler	Available in one strength only	Nasal Inhaler

When Prescribed: Vancenase nasal inhaler is prescribed for the relief of symptoms due to inflammation of nasal mucous membranes which respond poorly to conventional treatment.

Precautions and Warnings: Vancenase nasal inhaler should not be continued beyond 3 weeks in the absence of significant symptomatic improvement. Vancenase nasal inhaler should not be used in the presence of untreated localized infection involving the nasal mucosa. Patients should use Vancenase inhaler at regular intervals since its effectiveness depends on its regular use. Its use should be avoided by pregnant women and nursing mothers. Safety and effectiveness for children under 12 have not been established.

Side Effects and Adverse Reactions: Irritation, burning of nasal mucosa, sneezing attacks, local infection of the nose.

VANCERIL® (Schering Corporation)

Generic Name: Beclomethasone dipropionate

Dosage Form	Strength	Route
Inhaler	Available in one strength only	Oral inhalation

When Prescribed: Vanceril is prescribed to control asthma in patients who do not respond to other therapies.

Precautions and Warnings: The safe use of this drug in pregnancy and by nursing mothers has not been established.

Side Effects and Adverse Reactions: Oral infections, hoarseness, dry mouth, breathing difficulties, rash.

VASOCIDIN® (Cooper Vision Pharmaceuticals Inc.)

Generic Name: Sulfacetamide sodium, prednisolone sodium phosphate

Dosage Form	Strength	Route
Ophthalmic (eye) Solution	Available in one strength only	Eye Drops

When Prescribed: Vasocidin is a combination of an antiinfective and a steroid. It is prescribed for inflammatory ocular (eye) conditions associated with infection.

Precautions and Warnings: If inflammation or pain persists longer than 48 hours or becomes aggravated, the patient should be advised to discontinue using the medication and consult his physician. To prevent contamination, care should be taken to avoid touching dropper tip to eyelids or any other surface. Vasocidin should be used during pregnancy only if clearly needed. Caution should be exercised when Vasocidin is administered to a nursing mother. Safety and effectiveness for children under 6 have not been established.

Side Effects and Adverse Reactions: Prolonged use of Vasocidin may result in glaucoma with damage to optic nerve; development of secondary infection; delayed wound healing; stinging, burning, and irritation of the eye.

VASOTEC® (Merck Sharp and Dohme)

Generic Name: Enalapril maleate

Dosage Form	Strength	Route
Tablet	5 mg	Oral
	10 mg	Oral

When Prescribed: Vasotec is prescribed for treatment of high blood pressure.

Precautions and Warnings: If any abnormality occurs on face and/or throat, your physician should be informed immediately. Vasotec is a potent drug and it may decrease blood pressure below normal. Therefore, a patient may get dizzy while changing his or her position (from lying down to getting up). If this happens, inform your physician. The safe use of this drug by children has not been established.

Side Effects and Adverse Reactions: Headache, dizziness, fatigue, diarrhea, rash, lower blood pressure than considered normal, cough, nausea.

V-CILLIN K® (Eli Lilly and Company)

Generic Name: Potassium phenoxymethyl penicillin

Dosage Form	Strength	Route
Liquid	125 mg/5 cc	Oral
	250 mg/5 cc	Oral
Tablet	125 mg	Oral
	250 mg	Oral
	500 mg	Oral

When Prescribed: V-Cillin K is a form of penicillin which is prescribed for the treatment of mild to moderately severe infections.

Precautions and Warnings: The use of any penicillin should be discontinued and a physician consulted if any of the symptoms listed below appear.

Side Effects and Adverse Reactions: Nausea, vomiting, chest or stomach pains, diarrhea, changes in color/texture of oral membranes, skin rash, hives, chills, fever, swelling, pain in joints, fainting, superinfection by nonsusceptible organisms.

VELOSEF® (E. R. Squibb & Sons, Inc.)

Generic Name: Cephradine

Dosage Form	Strength	Route
Liquid	125 mg/5 ml	Oral
	250 mg/5 ml	
Capsule	250 mg	Oral
	500 mg	
Tablet	1000 mg	Oral

When Prescribed: Velosef is an antibiotic prescribed for a variety of infections, including those of the respiratory tract, the ear, the skin and the urinary tract.

Precautions and Warnings: The safe use of this drug in pregnancy and in nursing mothers has not been established. This drug can cause allergic reactions in people who are allergic to penicillin.

Side Effects and Adverse Reactions: Inflammation of the tongue, nausea, vomiting, diarrhea, loose stools, abdominal pain, heartburn, rash, itching, pain in the joints, dizziness, tightness in the chest, vaginal infections.

VENTOLIN® (Glaxo, Inc.)

Generic Name: Albuterol

Dosage Form	Strength	Route
Inhaler	Available in one strength only	Inhaled orally
Tablet	2 mg	Oral
	4 mg	

When Prescribed: Ventolin is prescribed to help improve breathing in conditions such as asthma and other respiratory disorders.

Precautions and Warnings: Do not exceed recommended dosage. The safe use of this drug in pregnancy has not been established. Ventolin is not recommended for use in children under 12 years of age.

Side Effects and Adverse Reactions: Heart flutters, rapid heartbeat, tremor, nausea, dizziness, heartburn, nervousness, chest or arm pain, vomiting, loss of balance, stimulation, headache, insomnia, unusual taste, drying or irritation of the mouth, nose or throat.

VERMOX® (Janssen Pharmaceutical, Inc.)

Generic Name: Mebendazole

Dosage Form	Strength	Route
Chewable tablet	100 mg	Oral

When Prescribed: Vermox is prescribed for the treatment of various worm infections.

Precautions and Warnings: This drug should not be taken by pregnant women. The tablet may be swallowed whole, chewed, or crushed and mixed with food.

Side Effects and Adverse Reactions: Abdominal pain, diarrhea.

VIBRAMYCIN® (Pfizer Laboratories Division)

Generic Name: Doxycycline hyclate

Dosage Form	Strength	Route
Capsule	50 mg	Oral
	100 mg	Oral
Liquid	25 mg/5 ml	Oral
Liquid	50 mg/5 ml	Oral

When Prescribed: Vibramycin is derived from tetracycline and is an antibiotic prescribed for a variety of infections.

Precautions and Warnings: Vibramycin should not be taken by people overly sensitive to tetracycline. If any of the side effects listed below occur, consult your physician immediately. This drug should not be taken by pregnant women, infants, or children under 8.

Side Effects and Adverse Reactions: Exaggerated sunburn, superinfection by nonsusceptible organisms, loss of appetite, nausea, vomiting, diarrhea, inflammation of the tongue, difficulty swallowing, stomach pains, inflammation of the bowel and genital region, skin rash, hives, swelling, fainting.

VIBRA-TABS® (Pfizer Laboratories Division)

Generic Name: Doxycycline hyclate

Dosage Form	Strength	Route
Film-coated tablet	100 mg	Oral

When Prescribed: Vibra-Tabs is derived from tetracycline and is an antibiotic prescribed for a variety of infections.

Precautions and Warnings: Vibra-Tabs should not be taken by people overly sensitive to tetracycline. This drug should not be taken by pregnant women, nursing mothers, or children under 8 years of age.

Side Effects and Adverse Reactions: Exaggerated sunburn, superinfection by non-susceptible organisms, loss of appetite, nausea, vomiting, diarrhea, inflammation of the tongue, difficulty swallowing, stomach pains, inflammation of the bowel and genital region, skin rash, hives, swelling, fainting.

VICODIN® (Knoll Pharmaceutical Company)

Generic Name: Hydrocodone bitartrate and acetaminophen

Dosage Form	Strength	Route
Tablet	Available in one strength only	Oral

When Prescribed: Vicodin is prescribed for the relief of moderate to moderately severe pain.

Precautions and Warnings: This drug can possibly be physically addictive. Psychological dependence and tolerance (a larger dose is necessary to produce the same effect) can also occur. Patients taking this drug may become drowsy. If so, you should not drive or operate dangerous machinery. Vicodin should not be taken with alcohol, tranquilizers, sleeping pills or sedatives unless specifically directed by your physician. The safe use of this drug during pregnancy, in nursing mothers and in children has not been established.

Side Effects and Adverse Reactions: Sedation, drowsiness, mental clouding, lethargy, impairment of mental and physical performance, anxiety, fear, mood changes, dizziness, depression, nausea, vomiting, urinary difficulties, depression of breathing.

VISKEN® (Sandoz Pharmaceuticals)

Generic Name: Pindolol

Dosage Form	Strength	Route
Tablet	5 mg	Oral
	10 mg	Oral

When Prescribed: Visken is prescribed for management of high blood pressure. It may be used alone or with other drugs.

Precautions and Warnings: Visken should not be used by pregnant or nursing women. Safety and effectiveness for children have not been established. It should not be used by patients with asthma or other lung diseases. Visken therapy should not be stopped abruptly.

Side Effects and Adverse Reactions: Anxiety, bizarre dreams, dizziness, fatigue, insomnia, nervousness, difficulty in breathing, edema, chest pain, muscle pain, joint pain, abdominal discomfort, nausea.

VISTARIL® (Pfizer Laboratories Division)

Generic Name: Hydroxyzine pamoate

Dosage Form	Strength	Route
Capsule	25 mg	Oral
	50 mg	Oral
	100 mg	Oral
Liquid	25 mg/5 ml	Oral

When Prescribed: Vistaril is an antihistamine prescribed for the relief of anxiety and tension which can result from a wide variety of emotional or physical reasons. Vistaril is well tolerated by most individuals; for this reason it is often prescribed for long-term use. Also used to prevent vomiting.

Precautions and Warnings: This drug is not recommended for use during early pregnancy. Vistaril should not be taken with alcohol, sleeping pills, sedatives or tranquilizers unless directed by your physician. If drowsiness occurs, you should not drive or operate dangerous machinery. Mothers should not nurse while taking Vistaril.

Side Effects and Adverse Reactions: Drowsiness, dryness of the mouth, tremors, convulsions.

VOLTAREN® (Ceigy)

Generic Name: Diclofenac Sodium

Dosage Form	Strength	Route
Tablet	25 mg	Oral
	50 mg	Oral
	75 mg	Oral

When Prescribed: Voltaren is prescribed for the relief of acute and chronic symptoms of arthritis. It is also prescribed for ankylosing spondylitis.

Precautions and Warnings: Voltaren can cause serious bleeding and ulceration of the GI tract. Minor GI irritation such as nausea, heartburn, gas and indigestion is common and usually occurs early in treatment. Liver damage may occur in patients receiving long-term treatment, skin rash, nausea, fatigue, lethargy, itching, jaundice (yellowing of skin and eyes), flulike symptoms and tenderness in right, upper body are signs of liver malfunctioning. Voltaren can cause allergic reactions such as swelling of eyelids, lips, pharynx and larynx, raised patches of skin, intense itching, asthma, bronchial spasms, and a fall in blood pressure. Voltaren should be used cautiously by patients suffering from heart failure, hypertension and other conditions causing fluid retention. Voltaren may cause kidney failure with the elderly, those suffering from kidney disorders, heart failure, liver disease, and those taking diuretics at greatest risk. Voltaren may cause aggravation of porphyria. Voltaren should be used with caution during pregnancy and should be avoided altogether during late pregnancy and by nursing mothers.

Side Effects and Adverse Reactions: Pep-

VōSoL HC OTIC® (Wallace Laboratories)

Generic Name: Acetic acid—nonaqueous, hydrocortisone

Dosage Form	Strength	Route
Liquid	Available in one strength only	Otic (ear) drops

When Prescribed: VōSoL HC Otic drops are prescribed for treatment of bacterial infection and inflammation of the external ear canal.

Precautions and Warnings: If irritation occurs during VōSoL HC Otic use, stop the medication immediately. The safe use of VōSoL HC Otic and other steroids during pregnancy has not been confirmed. Carefully remove all wax to allow VōSoL HC to contact the infected surface immediately.

Side Effects and Adverse Reactions: Sensitization or irritation of skin, superinfection by nonsusceptible organisms.

Voltaren-(Continued)

tic ulcer and upper intestinal bleeding, headache, dizziness, abdominal pain, constipation, diarrhea, indigestion, nausea, abdominal swelling, liver test abnormalities, gas, bloody diarrhea, hepatitis, jaundice, vomiting, inflammation of the mouth, asthma, heart failure, fluid retention, appetite change, eczema, drowsiness, depression, insomnia, anxiety, irritability, blurred vision, blind or dark spots, double vision, reversible hearing loss, heart attack, increased heart rate, chest pain, frequent urination, urination during the night, vaginal bleeding, blood in urine, impotence, lesions of the esoph-

WESTCORT® (Westwood Pharmaceutical Inc.)

Generic Name: Hydrocortisone valerate

Dosage Form	Strength	Route
Cream, Ointment	0.2%	Topical (apply directly to affected area)

When Prescribed: Westcort is prescribed for the relief of pain, itching, and inflammation caused by allergic reactions.

Precautions and Warnings: Westcort should not be used in the eyes. The treated skin should not be bandaged or otherwise covered or wrapped unless directed by the physician. Parents of pediatric patients should not use tight-fitting diapers or plastic pants on a child being treated in the diaper area. Westcort should not be used extensively or for prolonged periods by pregnant women. Caution should be exercised when Westcort is administered to a nursing mother. Chronic use of this product may interfere with the growth and development of children.

Side Effects and Adverse Reactions: Burning, itching, irritation, dryness, inflammation of hair follicles, secondary infection, miliaria.

WYGESIC® (Wyeth Laboratories)

Generic Name: Propoxyphene hydrochloride, acetaminophen

Dosage Form	Strength	Route
Tablet	Available in one strength only	Oral

When Prescribed: Wygesic is prescribed for the relief of mild to moderate pain.

Precautions and Warnings: This drug should not be taken with alcohol, sleeping pills, sedatives, or tranquilizers unless directed by your physician. If Wygesic makes you drowsy, you should not drive or operate dangerous machinery. The safe use of this drug in pregnancy has not been established. This drug should not be taken by children under the age of 12 or by nursing mothers. If this drug is taken in higher than recommended doses over a prolonged period of time, physical and/or psychological dependence can occur.

Side Effects and Adverse Reactions: Dizziness, sedation, nausea, vomiting, constipation, abdominal pain, skin rashes, lightheadedness, headache, weakness, euphoria, uneasiness, minor visual disturbances.

agus, shortness of breath, hyperventilation, hypoglycemia, numbness of extremities, convulsions, memory disturbances, tremor, tic, dimness of sight, night blindness, eye problems, excessive perspiration.

WYMOX® (Wyeth Laboratories)

Generic Name: Amoxicillin

Dosage Form	Strength	Route
Capsule	250 mg	Oral
	500 mg	Oral
Suspension	125 mg/5 ml (1 teaspoon)	Oral
	250 mg/5 ml (1 teaspoon)	Oral

When Prescribed: Wymox is a synthetic penicillin that is prescribed for a wide variety of infections.

Precautions and Warnings: Wymox should not be taken by people who are allergic to penicillin. The use of any penicillin should be discontinued and your physician notified if any of the side effects or reactions listed below appear.

Side Effects and Adverse Reactions: Nausea, vomiting, chest or stomach pains, diarrhea, skin rash, hives, chills, fever, swelling, pain in joints, fainting, superinfection by nonsusceptible organisms, anemia, bruising, indigestion, difficulty in breathing, wheezing.

XANAX® (The Upjohn Company)

Generic Name: Alprazolam

Dosage Form	Strength	Route
Tablets	0.25 mg	Oral
	0.50 mg	
	1.00 mg	

When Prescribed: Xanax is prescribed for the relief of anxiety and anxiety that often accompanies depression.

Precautions and Warnings: Xanax can produce physical and/or psychological dependence. Xanax should not be abruptly discontinued after prolonged use. This drug should not be taken with alcohol, tranquilizers, sleeping pills or sedatives unless directed by your physician. If you become drowsy while taking this medication, you should not drive or operate dangerous machinery. This drug should not be taken by pregnant women, nursing mothers or children under the age of 18.

Side Effects and Adverse Reactions: Drowsiness, lightheadedness, depression, headache, confusion, insomnia, nervousness, fainting, dizziness, restlessness, dry mouth, constipation, diarrhea, nausea, vomiting, increased salivation, rapid heartbeat, heart flutters, blurred vision, rigid limbs, tremor, allergic skin reactions, nasal congestion, change in body weight.

XYLOCAINE® (Astra Pharmaceutical Products)

Generic Name: Lidocaine

Dosage Form	Strength	Route
Ointment	5%	Topical (apply directly to affected area)
Oral Spray	10%	Topical

When Prescribed: Xylocaine is prescribed when local anesthesia is required, especially for the mucous membranes of the mouth.

Precautions and Warnings: Xylocaine should be used with great caution if there is a sepsis or trauma of the mucous membranes. If you are allergic to any other drug, inform your physician about the allergy before using Xylocaine. In pregnant women and nursing women, it should be used with great caution. Safety and effectiveness for children under 12 have not been established.

Side Effects and Adverse Reactions: Excitation, depression, lightheadedness, nervousness, euphoria, convulsions, drowsiness, ringing in the ears, confusion, dizziness, unconsciousness, respiratory depression, decrease in blood pressure, decrease in heart rate, cardiac arrest.

ZANTAC® (Glaxo)

Generic Name: Ranitidine hydrochloride

Dosage Form	Strength	Route
Tablet	150 mg	Oral
	300 mg	Oral

When Prescribed: Zantac is prescribed for the treatment of duodenal ulcers, gastric ulcers, and certain other disorders associated with increased acid secretion in the stomach. It acts by reducing acid secretion in the stomach.

Precautions and Warnings: Zantac is recommended only for short-term treatment of ulcers. For gastric ulcers, it is recommended for up to 6 weeks, and for duodenal ulcers, for up to 8 weeks only. Nursing mothers and children should not take this drug.

Side Effects and Adverse Reactions: Insomnia, confusion, constipation, diarrhea, abdominal discomfort/pain, enlargement of breasts in males.

ZAROXOLYN® (Pennwalt)

Generic Name: Metolazone

Dosage Form	Strength	Route
Tablet	2.5 mg	Oral
	5 mg	Oral
	10 mg	Oral

When Prescribed: Zaroxolyn is prescribed for the treatment of high blood pressure and for the treatment of water and salt retention resulting from congestive heart failure or kidney disease. It acts by helping the body to pass salt and water.

Precautions and Warnings: This drug should not be taken by nursing mothers.

Side Effects and Adverse Reactions: Constipation, fainting, dizziness, drowsiness, dryness of the mouth, fatigue, muscle weakness, cramps, weakness, restlessness, nausea, vomiting, loss of appetite, diarrhea, bloating, heartburn, yellowing of skin, loss of balance, headache, skin rash, hives, chest pains, chills, yellow appearance of or halo around objects, increased sensitivity to sunlight.

ZOVIRAX® (Burroughs Wellcome Company)

Generic Name: Acyclovir

Dosage Form	Strength	Route
Capsule	200 mg	Oral
Ointment	5%	Topical (apply directly to affected area)

When Prescribed: Zovirax capsule is prescribed for the treatment of initial episodes and management of recurrent episodes of genital herpes in certain patients. Zovirax ointment is only prescribed for the management of initial herpes genitalis.

Precautions and Warnings: Zovirax should be avoided during pregnancy and nursing. Educational material is provided to pharmacists and other health care professionals to give to patients. If you are using Zovirax capsules, ask your pharmacist to give you one of these. Zovirax ointment should not be used in the eyes. If you are using Zovirax ointment, the prescribed frequency of application and length of treatment should not be exceeded. A finger cot or rubber glove should be used when applying Zovirax to prevent transmission of infection to other persons.

Side Effects and Adverse Reactions: With short-term use of Zovirax capsules, you may experience nausea and vomiting frequently. Less frequent side effects are: dizziness, fatigue, anorexia, edema, skin rash, leg pain, medication taste, and sore throat. The most frequent side effect with long-term use of Zovirax is headache. Other side effects are diarrhea, nausea, vomiting, skin rash, muscle cramps, menstruation abnormality,

ZYLOPRIM® (Burroughs Wellcome Company)

Generic Name: Allopurinol

Dosage Form	Strength	Route
Tablet	100 mg	Oral
	300 mg	Oral

When Prescribed: Zyloprim is prescribed for management of signs and symptoms of gout. It is also given to patients who are receiving cancer therapy.

Precautions and Warnings: An increase in acute attacks of gout has been reported during the early stage of Zyloprim administration. A sufficient amount of fluid intake is necessary with Zyloprim therapy. First sign of skin rash should be reported to the physician.

Side Effects and Adverse Reactions: Diarrhea, nausea, skin rash, fever, headache, abdominal pain, dyspepsia.

Zovirax-(Continued)

accelerated hair loss, depression. Patients may experience discomfort upon application of the ointment. Other side effects are inflammation and rash.

DRUG CATEGORY INDEX

DRUG NAME INDEX